Virtual Clinical Excursions—Med

for

Ignatavicius, Workman, and Rebar:
Medical-Surgical Nursing:
Concepts for Interprofessional Collaborative Care,
9th Edition

Virtual Clinical Excursions—Medical-Surgical

for

Ignatavicius, Workman, and Rebar: Medical-Surgical Nursing: Concepts for Interprofessional Collaborative Care, 9th Edition

prepared by

Sandra J. Bleza, MSN, RN, CNE, CHSE
Clinical Assistant Professor
College of Nursing and Health Professions
Valparaiso University
Valparaiso, Indiana

software developed by

Wolfsong Informatics, LLC
Tucson, Arizona

ELSEVIER

ELSEVIER

3251 Riverport Lane
Maryland Heights, Missouri 63043

VIRTUAL CLINICAL EXCURSIONS—MEDICAL-SURGICAL FOR
IGNATAVICIUS, WORKMAN, AND REBAR: MEDICAL-SURGICAL NURSING:
CONCEPTS FOR INTERPROFESSIONAL COLLABORATIVE CARE,
NINTH EDITION

ISBN: 978-0-323-46168-9

Notice

Knowledge and best practice in this field are constantly changing. As new research and experience broaden our understanding, changes in research methods, professional practices, or medical treatment may become necessary.

Practitioners and researchers must always rely on their own experience and knowledge in evaluating and using any information, methods, compounds, or experiments described herein. In using such information or methods they should be mindful of their own safety and the safety of others, including parties for whom they have a professional responsibility.

With respect to any drug or pharmaceutical products identified, readers are advised to check the most current information provided (i) on procedures featured or (ii) by the manufacturer of each product to be administered, to verify the recommended dose or formula, the method and duration of administration, and contraindications. It is the responsibility of practitioners, relying on their own experience and knowledge of their patients, to make diagnoses, to determine dosages and the best treatment for each individual patient, and to take all appropriate safety precautions.

To the fullest extent of the law, neither the Publisher nor the authors, contributors, or editors, assume any liability for any injury and/or damage to persons or property as a matter of products liability, negligence or otherwise, or from any use or operation of any methods, products, instructions, or ideas contained in the material herein.

ISBN: 978-0-323-46168-9

Printed in the United States of America

Last digit is the print number: 9 8 7 6 5 4 3 2 1

Textbook

Donna D. Ignatavicius, MS, RN, CNE, ANEF
Speaker and Curriculum Consultant for Academic Nursing Programs
Founder, Boot Camp for Nurse Educators
President, DI Associates, Inc.
Littleton, Colorado

M. Linda Workman, PhD, RN, FAAN
Author and Consultant
Cincinnati, Ohio

Cherie R. Rebar, PhD, MBA, RN, COI
Professor of Nursing
Wittenberg University
Springfield, Ohio

Table of Contents
Virtual Clinical Excursions Workbook

Table of Contents
Ignatavicius, Workman, and Rebar:
Medical-Surgical Nursing:
Concepts for Interprofessional Collaborative Care, 9th Edition

GETTING SET UP WITH VCE ONLINE ————————————————

The product you have purchased is part of the Evolve Learning System. Please read the following information thoroughly to get started.

■ HOW TO ACCESS YOUR VCE RESOURCES ON EVOLVE

There are two ways to access your VCE Resources on Evolve:

1. If your instructor has enrolled you in your VCE Evolve Resources, you will receive an email with your registration details.

2. If your instructor has asked you to self-enroll in your VCE Evolve Resources, he or she will provide you with your Course ID (for example, 1479_jdoe73_0001). You will then need to follow the instructions at https://evolve.elsevier.com/cs/studentEnroll.html.

■ HOW TO ACCESS THE ONLINE VIRTUAL HOSPITAL

The online virtual hospital is available through the Evolve VCE Resources. There is no software to download or install: the online virtual hospital runs within your Internet browser, using a pop-up window.

■ TECHNICAL REQUIREMENTS

- Broadband connection (DSL or cable)
- 1024 x 768 screen resolution
- Mozilla Firefox 18.0, Internet Explorer 9.0, Google Chrome, or Safari 5 (or higher)
  Note: Pop-up blocking software/settings must be disabled.
- Adobe Acrobat Reader
- Additional technical requirements available at http://evolvesupport.elsevier.com

■ HOW TO ACCESS THE WORKBOOK

There are two ways to access the workbook portion of *Virtual Clinical Excursions:*

1. Print workbook
2. An electronic version of the workbook, available within the VCE Evolve Resources

■ TECHNICAL SUPPORT

Technical support for *Virtual Clinical Excursions* is available by visiting the Technical Support Center at http://evolvesupport.elsevier.com or by calling 1-800-222-9570 inside the United States and Canada.

Trademarks: Windows® and Macintosh® are registered trademarks.

A QUICK TOUR

Welcome to *Virtual Clinical Excursions—Medical-Surgical*, a virtual hospital setting in which you can work with multiple complex patient simulations and also learn to access and evaluate the information resources that are essential for high-quality patient care. The virtual hospital, Pacific View Regional Hospital, has realistic architecture and access to patient rooms, a Nurses' Station, and a Medication Room.

■ BEFORE YOU START

Make sure you have your textbook nearby when you use *Virtual Clinical Excursions*. You will want to consult topic areas in your textbook frequently while working with the virtual hospital and workbook.

■ HOW TO SIGN IN

- Enter your name on the Student Nurse identification badge.
- Now choose one of the four periods of care in which to work. In Periods of Care 1 through 3, you can actively engage in patient assessment, entry of data in the electronic patient record (EPR), and medication administration. Period of Care 4 presents the day in review. Highlight and click the appropriate period of care. (For this quick tour, choose **Period of Care 1: 0730-0815**.)
- This takes you to the Patient List screen (see the *How to Select a Patient* section below). Only the patients on the Medical-Surgical Floor are available. Note that the virtual time is provided in the box at the lower left corner of the screen (0730, because we chose Period of Care 1).

Note: If you choose to work during Period of Care 4: 1900-2000, the Patient List screen is skipped because you are not able to visit patients or administer medications during the shift. Instead, you are taken directly to the Nurses' Station, where the records of all the patients on the floor are available for your review.

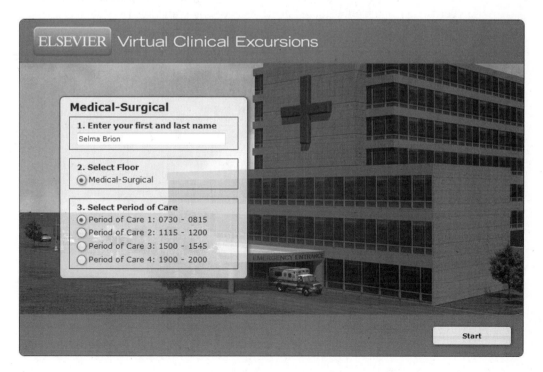

■ PATIENT LIST

MEDICAL-SURGICAL UNIT

Harry George (Room 401)
Osteomyelitis—A 54-year-old Caucasian male admitted from a homeless shelter with an infected leg. He has complications of type 2 diabetes mellitus, alcohol abuse, nicotine addiction, poor pain control, and complex psychosocial issues.

Jacquline Catanazaro (Room 402)
Asthma—A 45-year-old Caucasian female admitted with an acute asthma exacerbation and suspected pneumonia. She has complications of chronic schizophrenia, noncompliance with medication therapy, obesity, and herniated disc.

Piya Jordan (Room 403)
Bowel obstruction—A 68-year-old Asian female admitted with a colon mass and suspected adenocarcinoma. She undergoes a right hemicolectomy. This patient's complications include atrial fibrillation, hypokalemia, and symptoms of meperidine toxicity.

Clarence Hughes (Room 404)
Degenerative joint disease—A 73-year-old African-American male admitted for a left total knee replacement. His preparations for discharge are complicated by the development of a pulmonary embolus and the need for ongoing intravenous therapy.

Pablo Rodriguez (Room 405)
Metastatic lung carcinoma—A 71-year-old Hispanic male admitted with symptoms of dehydration and malnutrition. He has chronic pain secondary to multiple subcutaneous skin nodules and psychosocial concerns related to family issues with his approaching death.

Patricia Newman (Room 406)
Pneumonia—A 61-year-old Caucasian female admitted with worsening pulmonary function and an acute respiratory infection. Her chronic emphysema is complicated by heavy smoking, hypertension, and malnutrition. She needs access to community resources such as a smoking cessation program and meal assistance.

■ HOW TO SELECT A PATIENT

- You can choose one or more patients to work with from the Patient List by checking the box to the left of the patient name(s). For this quick tour, select Piya Jordan and Pablo Rodriguez. (In order to receive a scorecard for a patient, the patient must be selected before proceeding to the Nurses' Station.)
- Click on **Get Report** to the right of the medical records number (MRN) to view a summary of the patient's care during the 12-hour period before your arrival on the unit.
- After reviewing the report, click on **Go to Nurses' Station** in the right lower corner to begin your care. (*Note:* If you have been assigned to care for multiple patients, you can click on **Return to Patient List** to select and review the report for each additional patient before going to the Nurses' Station.)

Note: Even though the Patient List is initially skipped when you sign in to work for Period of Care 4, you can still access this screen if you wish to review the shift report for any of the patients. To do so, simply click on **Patient List** near the top left corner of the Nurses' Station (or click on the clipboard to the left of the Kardex). Then click on **Get Report** for the patient(s) whose care you are reviewing. This may be done during any period of care.

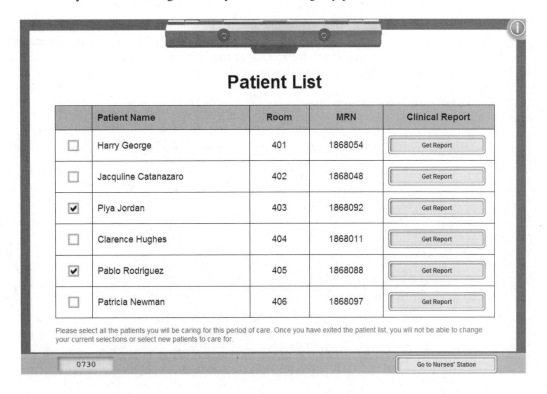

Patient List

	Patient Name	Room	MRN	Clinical Report
☐	Harry George	401	1868054	Get Report
☐	Jacquline Catanazaro	402	1868048	Get Report
☑	Piya Jordan	403	1868092	Get Report
☐	Clarence Hughes	404	1868011	Get Report
☑	Pablo Rodriguez	405	1868088	Get Report
☐	Patricia Newman	406	1868097	Get Report

Please select all the patients you will be caring for this period of care. Once you have exited the patient list, you will not be able to change your current selections or select new patients to care for.

0730   Go to Nurses' Station

■ HOW TO FIND A PATIENT'S RECORDS

NURSES' STATION

Within the Nurses' Station, you will see:

1. A clipboard that contains the patient list for that floor.
2. A chart rack with patient charts labeled by room number, a notebook labeled Kardex, and a notebook labeled MAR (Medication Administration Record).
3. A desktop computer with access to the Electronic Patient Record (EPR).
4. A tool bar across the top of the screen that can also be used to access the Patient List, EPR, Chart, MAR, and Kardex. This tool bar is also accessible from each patient's room.
5. A Drug Guide containing information about the medications you are able to administer to your patients.
6. A Laboratory Guide containing normal value ranges for all laboratory tests you may come across in the virtual patient hospital.
7. A tool bar across the bottom of the screen that can be used to access the Floor Map, patient rooms, Medication Room, and Drug Guide.

As you run your cursor over an item, it will be highlighted. To select, simply click on the item. As you use these resources, you will always be able to return to the Nurses' Station by clicking on the **Return to Nurses' Station** bar located in the right lower corner of your screen.

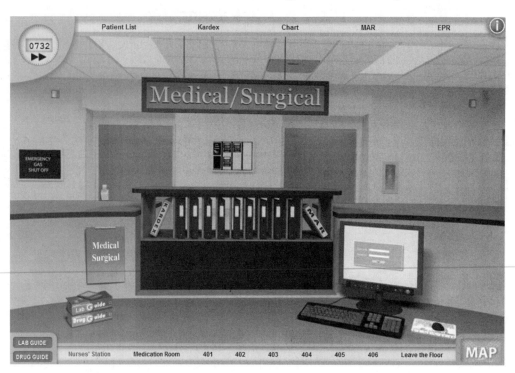

MEDICATION ADMINISTRATION RECORD (MAR)

The MAR icon located on the tool bar at the top of your screen accesses current 24-hour medications for each patient. Click on the icon and the MAR will open. (*Note:* You can also access the MAR by clicking on the MAR notebook on the far right side of the book rack in the center of the screen.) Within the MAR, tabs on the right side of the screen allow you to select patients by room number. Be careful to make sure you select the correct tab number for *your* patient rather than simply reading the first record that appears after the MAR opens. Each MAR sheet lists the following:

- Medications
- Route and dosage of each medication
- Times of administration of each medication

Note: The MAR changes each day. Expired MARs are stored in the patients' charts.

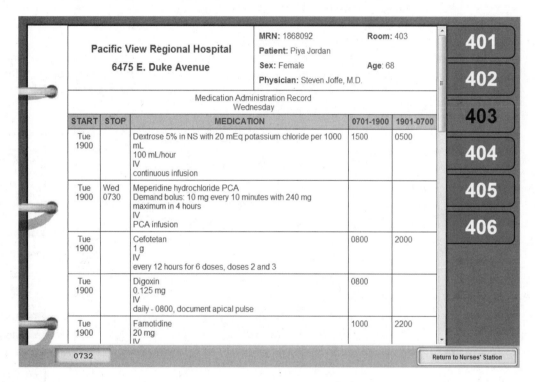

Pacific View Regional Hospital
6475 E. Duke Avenue

MRN: 1868092	Room: 403
Patient: Piya Jordan	
Sex: Female	Age: 68
Physician: Steven Joffe, M.D.	

Medication Administration Record
Wednesday

START	STOP	MEDICATION	0701-1900	1901-0700
Tue 1900		Dextrose 5% in NS with 20 mEq potassium chloride per 1000 mL 100 mL/hour IV continuous infusion	1500	0500
Tue 1900	Wed 0730	Meperidine hydrochloride PCA Demand bolus: 10 mg every 10 minutes with 240 mg maximum in 4 hours IV PCA infusion		
Tue 1900		Cefotetan 1 g IV every 12 hours for 6 doses, doses 2 and 3	0800	2000
Tue 1900		Digoxin 0.125 mg IV daily - 0800, document apical pulse	0800	
Tue 1900		Famotidine 20 mg IV	1000	2200

Tabs: 401, 402, 403, 404, 405, 406

0732

Return to Nurses' Station

CHARTS

To access patient charts, either click on the **Chart** icon at the top of your screen or anywhere within the chart rack in the center of the Nurses' Station screen. When the close-up view appears, the individual charts are labeled by room number. To open a chart, click on the room number of the patient whose chart you wish to review. The patient's name and allergies will appear on the left side of the screen, along with a list of tabs on the right side of the screen, allowing you to view the following data:

- Allergies
- Physician's Orders
- Physician's Notes
- Nurse's Notes
- Laboratory Reports
- Diagnostic Reports
- Surgical Reports
- Consultations

- Patient Education
- History and Physical
- Nursing Admission
- Expired MARs
- Consents
- Mental Health
- Admissions
- Emergency Department

Information appears in real time. The entries are in reverse chronologic order, so use the down arrow at the right side of each chart page to scroll down to view previous entries. Flip from tab to tab to view multiple data fields or click on **Return to Nurses' Station** in the lower right corner of the screen to exit the chart.

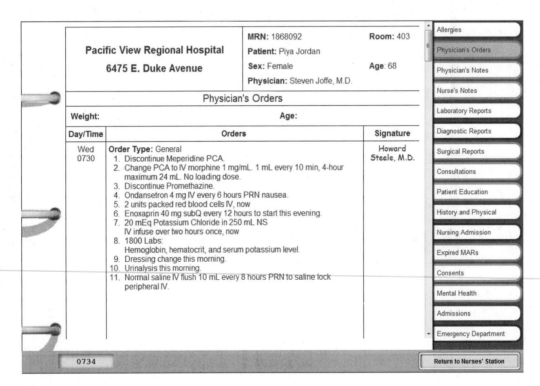

ELECTRONIC PATIENT RECORD (EPR)

The EPR can be accessed from the computer in the Nurses' Station or from the EPR icon located in the tool bar at the top of your screen. To access a patient's EPR:
- Click on either the computer screen or the **EPR** icon.
- Your username and password are automatically filled in.
- Click on **Login** to enter the EPR.
- *Note:* Like the MAR, the EPR is arranged numerically. Thus when you enter, you are initially shown the records of the patient in the lowest room number on the floor. To view the correct data for *your* patient, remember to select the correct room number, using the drop-down menu for the Patient field at the top left corner of the screen.

The EPR used in Pacific View Regional Hospital represents a composite of commercial versions being used in hospitals. You can access the EPR:
- to review existing data for a patient (by room number).
- to enter data you collect while working with a patient.

The EPR is updated daily, so no matter what day or part of a shift you are working, there will be a current EPR with the patient's data from the past days of the current hospital stay. This type of simulated EPR allows you to examine how data for different attributes have changed over time, as well as to examine data for all of a patient's attributes at a particular time. The EPR is fully functional (as it is in a real-life hospital). You can enter such data as blood pressure, breath sounds, and certain treatments. The EPR will not, however, allow you to enter data for a previous time period. Use the arrows at the bottom of the screen to move forward and backward in time.

Patient Room: 403	Category: Vital Signs			Electronic Patient Records
Name: Piya Jordan	Wed 0700	Wed 0715	Wed 0731	Code Meanings
PAIN: LOCATION	OS			
PAIN: RATING	5			
PAIN: CHARACTERISTICS	C	NN		
PAIN: VOCAL CUES	VC3			
PAIN: FACIAL CUES	FC1			
PAIN: BODILY CUES				
PAIN: SYSTEM CUES				
PAIN: FUNCTIONAL EFFECTS				
PAIN: PREDISPOSING FACTORS				
PAIN: RELIEVING FACTORS				
PCA				
TEMPERATURE (F)	P			
TEMPERATURE (C)	99.6			
MODE OF MEASUREMENT				
SYSTOLIC PRESSURE	Ty			
DIASTOLIC PRESSURE	110	149		
BP MODE OF MEASUREMENT	70	94		
HEART RATE	NIBP	NIBP		
RESPIRATORY RATE	104	152		
SpO2 (%)	18	32		
BLOOD GLUCOSE	95	85		
WEIGHT				
HEIGHT				

0731   Return to Nurses' Station

At the top of the EPR screen, you can choose patients by their room numbers. In addition, you have access to 17 different categories of patient data. To change patients or data categories, click the down arrow to the right of the room number or category.

The categories of patient data in the EPR are as follows:

- Vital Signs
- Respiratory
- Cardiovascular
- Neurologic
- Gastrointestinal
- Excretory
- Musculoskeletal
- Integumentary
- Reproductive
- Psychosocial
- Wounds and Drains
- Activity
- Hygiene and Comfort
- Safety
- Nutrition
- IV
- Intake and Output

Remember, each hospital selects its own codes. The codes used in the EPR at Pacific View Regional Hospital may be different from ones you have seen in your clinical rotations. Take some time to acquaint yourself with the codes. Within the Vital Signs category, click on any item in the left column (e.g., Pain: Characteristics). In the far-right column, you will see a list of code meanings for the possible findings and/or descriptors for that assessment area.

You will use the codes to record the data you collect as you work with patients. Click on the box in the last time column to the right of any item and wait for the code meanings applicable to that entry to appear. Select the appropriate code to describe your assessment findings and type it in the box. (*Note:* If no cursor appears within the box, click on the box again until the blue shading disappears and the blinking cursor appears.) Once the data are typed in this box, they are entered into the patient's record for this period of care only.

To leave the EPR, click on **Exit EPR** in the bottom right corner of the screen.

■ VISITING A PATIENT

From the Nurses' Station, click on the room number of the patient you wish to visit (in the tool bar at the bottom of your screen). Once you are inside the room, you will see a still photo of your patient in the top left corner. To verify that this is the correct patient, click on the **Check Armband** icon to the right of the photo. The patient's identification data will appear. If you click on **Check Allergies** (the next icon to the right), a list of the patient's allergies (if any) will replace the photo.

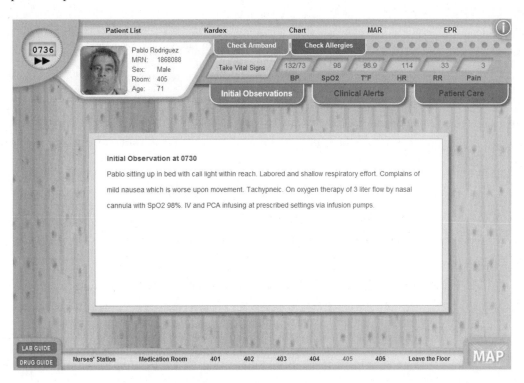

Also located in the patient's room are multiple icons you can use to assess the patient or the patient's medications. A virtual clock is provided in the upper left corner of the room to monitor your progress in real time. (*Note:* The fast-forward icon within the virtual clock will advance the time by 2-minute intervals when clicked.)

- The tool bar across the top of the screen allows you to check the **Patient List**, access the **EPR** to check or enter data, and view the patient's **Chart**, **MAR**, or **Kardex**.

- The **Take Vital Signs** icon allows you to measure the patient's up-to-the-minute blood pressure, oxygen saturation, temperature, heart rate, respiratory rate, and pain level.

- Each time you enter a patient's room, you are given an Initial Observation report to review (in the text box under the patient's photo). These notes are provided to give you a "look" at the patient as if you had just stepped into the room. You can also click on the **Initial Observations** icon to return to this box from other views within the patient's room. To the right of this icon is **Clinical Alerts**, a resource that allows you to make decisions about priority medication interventions based on emerging data collected in real time. Check this screen throughout your period of care to avoid missing critical information related to recently ordered or STAT medications.

- Clicking on **Patient Care** opens up three specific learning environments within the patient room: **Physical Assessment**, **Nurse-Client Interactions**, and **Medication Administration**.

- To perform a **Physical Assessment**, choose a body area (such as **Head & Neck**) from the column of yellow buttons. This activates a list of system subcategories for that body area (e.g., see **Sensory**, **Neurologic**, etc. in the green boxes). After you select the system you wish to evaluate, a brief description of the assessment findings will appear in a box to the right. A still photo provides a "snapshot" of how an assessment of this area might be done or what the finding might look like. For every body area, you can also click on **Equipment** on the right side of the screen.

- To the right of the Physical Assessment icon is **Nurse-Client Interactions**. Clicking on this icon will reveal the times and titles of any videos available for viewing. (*Note:* If the video you wish to see is not listed, this means you have not yet reached the correct virtual time to view that video. Check the virtual clock; you may return to access the video once its designated time has occurred—as long as you do so within the same period of care. Or you can click on the fast-forward icon within the virtual clock to advance the time by 2-minute intervals. You will then need to click again on **Patient Care** and **Nurse-Client Interactions** to refresh the screen.) To view a listed video, click on the white arrow to the right of the video title. Use the control buttons below the video to start, stop, pause, rewind, or fast-forward the action or to mute the sound.

- **Medication Administration** is the pathway that allows you to review and administer medications to a patient after you have prepared them in the Medication Room. This process is also addressed further in the *How to Prepare Medications* section below and in *Medications* in **A Detailed Tour**. For additional hands-on practice, see *Reducing Medication Errors* below **A Quick Tour** and **A Detailed Tour** in your resources.

■ HOW TO CHANGE PATIENTS OR CHANGE PERIODS OF CARE

How to Change Patients or Periods of Care: To change patients, simply click on the new patient's room number. (You cannot receive a scorecard for a new patient, however, unless you have already selected that patient on the Patient List screen.) To change to a new period of care or to restart the virtual clock, click on **Leave the Floor** and then on **Restart the Program**.

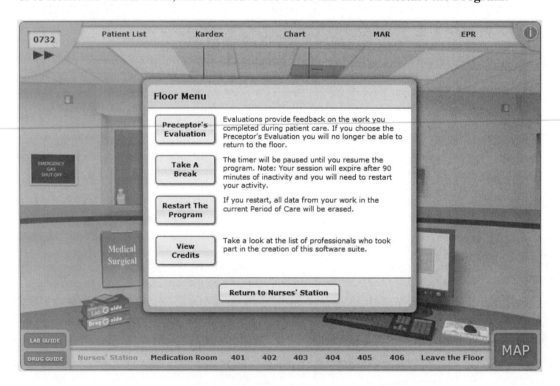

■ HOW TO PREPARE MEDICATIONS

From the Nurses' Station or the patient's room, you can access the Medication Room by clicking on the icon in the tool bar at the bottom of your screen to the left of the patient room numbers.

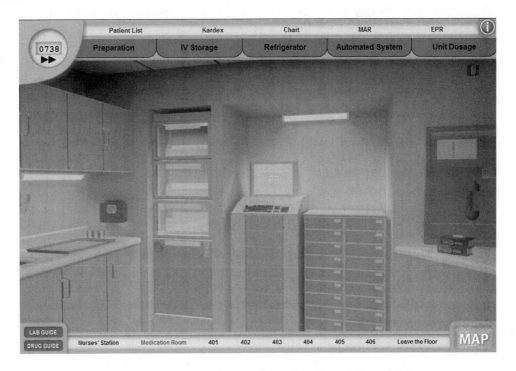

In the Medication Room you have access to the following (from left to right):

- A preparation area is located on the counter under the cabinets. To begin the medication preparation process, click on the tray on the counter or click on the **Preparation** icon at the top of the screen. The next screen leads you through a specific sequence (called the Preparation Wizard) to prepare medications one at a time for administration to a patient. However, no medication has been selected at this time. We will do this while working with a patient in **A Detailed Tour**. To exit this screen, click on **View Medication Room**.

- To the right of the cabinets (and above the refrigerator), IV storage bins are provided. Click on the bins themselves or on the **IV Storage** icon at the top of the screen. The bins are labeled **Microinfusion**, **Small Volume**, and **Large Volume**. Click on an individual bin to see a list of its contents. If you needed to prepare an IV medication at this time, you could click on the medication and its label would appear to the right under the patient's name. (*Note:* You can **Open** and **Close** any medication label by clicking the appropriate icon.) Next, you would click **Put Medication on Tray**. If you ever change your mind or decide that you have put the incorrect medication on the tray, you can reverse your actions by highlighting the medication on the tray and then clicking **Put Medication in Bin**. Click **Close Bin** in the right bottom corner to exit. **View Medication Room** brings you back to a full view of the entire room.

- A refrigerator is located under the IV storage bins to hold any medications that must be stored below room temperature. Click on the refrigerator door or on the **Refrigerator** icon at the top of the screen. Then click on the close-up view of the door to access the medications. When you are finished, click **Close Door** and then **View Medication Room**.

- To prepare controlled substances, click the **Automated System** icon at the top of the screen or click the computer monitor located to the right of the IV storage bins. A login screen will appear; your name and password are automatically filled in. Click **Login**. Select the patient for whom you wish to access medications; then select the correct medication drawer to open (they are stored alphabetically). Click **Open Drawer**, highlight the proper medication, and choose **Put Medication on Tray**. When you are finished, click **Close Drawer** and then **View Medication Room**.

- Next to the Automated System is a set of drawers identified by patient room number. To access these, click on the drawers or on the **Unit Dosage** icon at the top of the screen. This provides a close-up view of the drawers. To open a drawer, click on the room number of the patient you are working with. Next, click on the medication you would like to prepare for the patient, and a label will appear, listing the medication strength, units, and dosage per unit. To exit, click **Close Drawer**; then click **View Medication Room**.

At any time, you can learn about a medication you wish to prepare for a patient by clicking on the **Drug** icon in the bottom left corner of the medication room screen or by clicking the **Drug Guide** book on the counter to the right of the unit dosage drawers. The **Drug Guide** provides information about the medications commonly included in nursing drug handbooks. Nutritional supplements and maintenance intravenous fluid preparations are not included. Highlight a medication in the alphabetical list; relevant information about the drug will appear in the screen below. To exit, click **Return to Medication Room**.

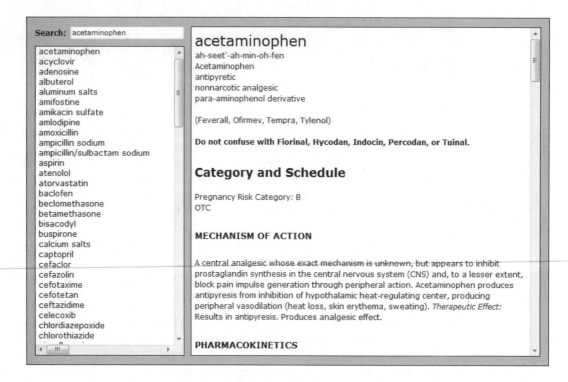

To access the MAR from the Medication Room and to review the medications ordered for a patient, click on the **MAR** icon located in the tool bar at the top of your screen and then click on the correct tab for your patient's room number. You may also click the **Review MAR** icon in the tool bar at the bottom of your screen from inside each medication storage area.

After you have chosen and prepared medications, go to the patient's room to administer them by clicking on the room number in the bottom tool bar. Inside the patient's room, click **Patient Care** and then **Medication Administration** and follow the proper administration sequence.

■ PRECEPTOR'S EVALUATIONS

When you have finished a session, click on **Leave the Floor** to go to the Floor Menu. At this point, you can click on the top icon (**Look at Your Preceptor's Evaluation**) to receive a score-card that provides feedback on the work you completed during patient care.

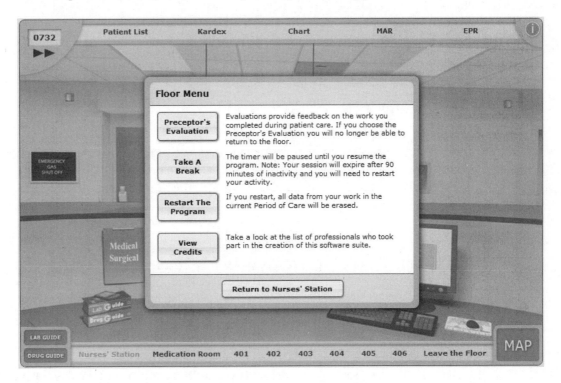

Evaluations are available for each patient you selected when you signed in for the current period of care. Click on the **Medication Scorecard** icon to see an example.

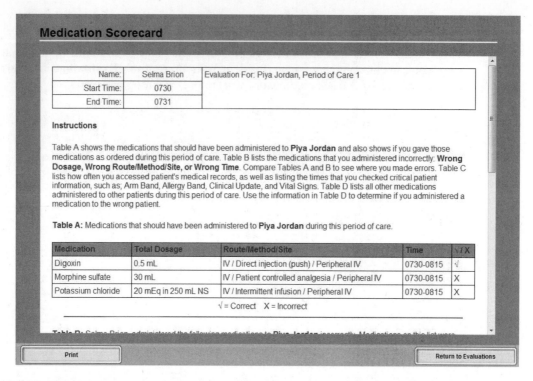

The scorecard compares the medications you administered to a patient during a period of care with what should have been administered. Table A lists the correct medications. Table B lists any medications that were administered incorrectly.

Remember, not every medication listed on the MAR should necessarily be given. For example, a patient might have an allergy to a drug that was ordered, or a medication might have been improperly transcribed to the MAR. Predetermined medication "errors" embedded within the program challenge you to exercise critical thinking skills and professional judgment when deciding to administer a medication, just as you would in a real hospital. Use all your available resources, such as the patient's chart and the MAR, to make your decision.

Table C lists the resources that were available to assist you in medication administration. It also documents whether and when you accessed these resources. For example, did you check the patient armband or perform a check of vital signs? If so, when?

You can click **Print** to get a copy of this report if needed. When you have finished reviewing the scorecard, click **Return to Evaluations** and then **Return to Menu**.

■ FLOOR MAP

To get a general sense of your location within the hospital, you can click on the **Map** icon found in the lower right corner of most of the screens in the *Virtual Clinical Excursions—Medical-Surgical* program. (*Note:* If you are following this quick tour step by step, you will need to **Restart the Program** from the Floor Menu, sign in again, and go to the Nurses' Station to access the map.) When you click the **Map** icon, a floor map appears, showing the layout of the floor you are currently on, as well as a directory of the patients and services on that floor. As you move your cursor over the directory list, the location of each room is highlighted on the map (and vice versa). The floor map can be accessed from the Nurses' Station, Medication Room, and each patient's room.

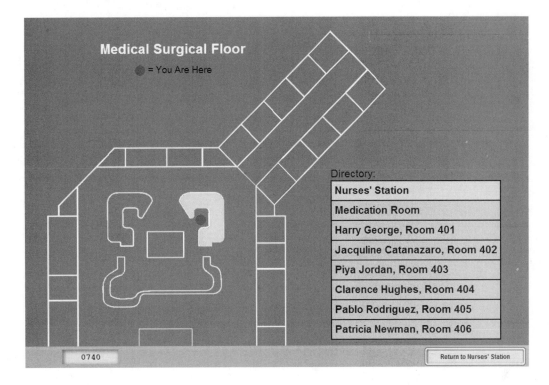

A DETAILED TOUR

If you wish to more thoroughly understand the capabilities of *Virtual Clinical Excursions—Medical-Surgical*, take a detailed tour by completing the following section. During this tour, we will work with a specific patient to introduce you to all the different components and learning opportunities available within the software.

■ WORKING WITH A PATIENT

Sign in for Period of Care 1 (0730-0815). From the Patient List, select Piya Jordan and Pablo Rodriguez; however, do not go to the Nurses' Station yet.

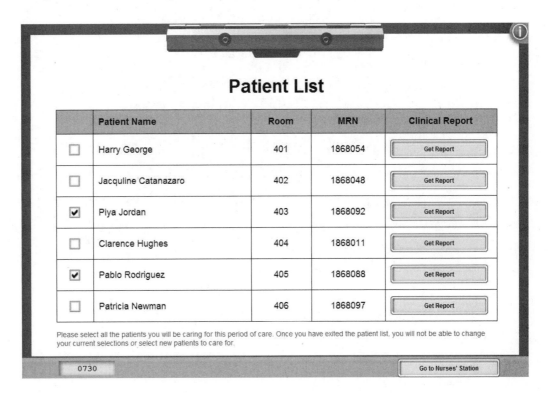

Patient List

	Patient Name	Room	MRN	Clinical Report
☐	Harry George	401	1868054	Get Report
☐	Jacquline Catanazaro	402	1868048	Get Report
☑	Piya Jordan	403	1868092	Get Report
☐	Clarence Hughes	404	1868011	Get Report
☑	Pablo Rodriguez	405	1868088	Get Report
☐	Patricia Newman	406	1868097	Get Report

Please select all the patients you will be caring for this period of care. Once you have exited the patient list, you will not be able to change your current selections or select new patients to care for.

0730   Go to Nurses' Station

■ REPORT

In hospitals, when one shift ends and another begins, the outgoing nurse who attended a patient will give a verbal and sometimes a written summary of that patient's condition to the incoming nurse who will assume care for the patient. This summary is called a report and is an important source of data to provide an overview of a patient. Your first task is to get the clinical report on Piya Jordan. To do this, click **Get Report** in the far right column in this patient's row. From a brief review of this summary, identify the problems and areas of concern that you will need to address for this patient.

When you have finished noting any areas of concern, click **Go to Nurses' Station**.

■ **CHARTS**

You can access Piya Jordan's chart from the Nurses' Station or from the patient's room (403).
From the Nurses' Station, click on the chart rack or on the **Chart** icon in the tool bar at the top
of your screen. Next, click on the chart labeled **403** to open the medical record for Piya Jordan.
Click on the **Emergency Department** tab to view a record of why this patient was admitted.

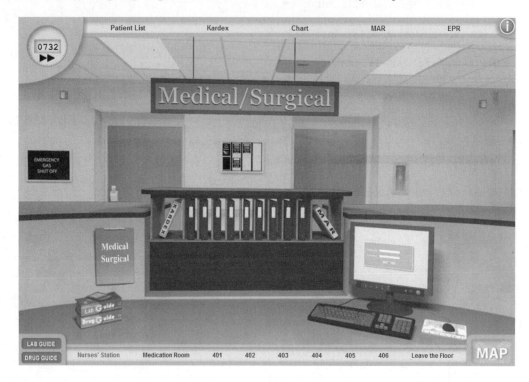

How many days has Piya Jordan been in the hospital?

What tests were done upon her arrival in the Emergency Department and why?

What was her reason for admission?

You should also click on **Diagnostic Reports** to learn what additional tests or procedures were
performed and when. Finally, review the **Nursing Admission** and **History and Physical** to
learn about the health history of this patient. When you are done reviewing the chart, click
Return to Nurses' Station.

■ MEDICATIONS

Open the Medication Administration Record (MAR) by clicking on the **MAR** icon in the tool bar at the top of your screen. *Remember:* The MAR automatically opens to the first occupied room number on the floor—which is not necessarily your patient's room number! Because you need to access Piya Jordan's MAR, click on tab **403** (her room number). Always make sure you are giving the *Right Drug to the Right Patient!*

Examine the list of medications ordered for Piya Jordan. In the table below, list the medications that need to be given during this period of care (0730-0815). For each medication, note the dosage, route, and time to be given.

Time	Medication	Dosage	Route

Click on **Return to Nurses' Station**. Next, click on **403** on the bottom tool bar and then verify that you are indeed in Piya Jordan's room. Select **Clinical Alerts** (the icon to the right of Initial Observations) to check for any emerging data that might affect your medication administration priorities. Next, go to the patient's chart (click on the **Chart** icon; then click on **403**). When the chart opens, select the **Physician's Orders** tab.

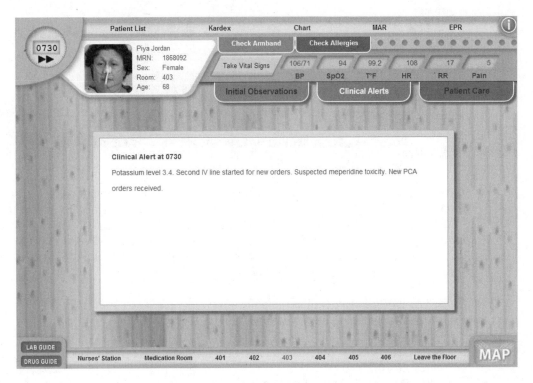

Review the orders. Have any new medications been ordered? Return to the MAR (click **Return to Room 403**; then click **MAR**). Verify that any new medications have been correctly transcribed to the MAR. Mistakes are sometimes made in the transcription process in the hospital setting, and it is sound practice to double-check any new order.

Are there any patient assessments you will need to perform before administering these medications? If so, return to Room 403 and click on **Patient Care** and then **Physical Assessment** to complete those assessments before proceeding.

Now click on the **Medication Room** icon in the tool bar at the bottom of your screen to locate and prepare the medications for Piya Jordan.

In the Medication Room, you must access the medications for Piya Jordan from the specific dispensing system in which each medication is stored. Locate each medication that needs to be given in this time period and click on **Put Medication on Tray** as appropriate. (*Hint:* Look in **Unit Dosage** drawer first.) When you are finished, click on **Close Drawer** and then on **View Medication Room**. Now click on the medication tray on the counter on the left side of the medication room screen to begin preparing the medications you have selected. (*Remember:* You can also click **Preparation** in the tool bar at the top of the screen.)

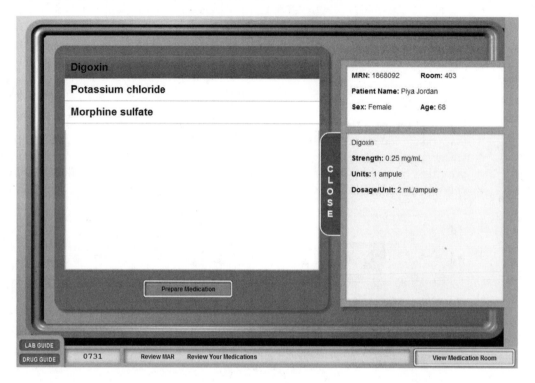

In the preparation area, you should see a list of the medications you put on the tray in the previous steps. Click on the first medication and then click **Prepare**. Follow the onscreen instructions of the Preparation Wizard, providing any data requested. As an example, let's follow the preparation process for digoxin, one of the medications due to be administered to Piya Jordan during this period of care. To begin, click to select **Digoxin**; then click **Prepare**. Now work through the Preparation Wizard sequence as detailed below:

> Amount of medication in the ampule: 2 mL.
> Enter the amount of medication you will draw up into a syringe: <u>**0.5**</u> mL.
> Click **Next**.
> Select the patient you wish to set aside the medication for: **Room 403, Piya Jordan**.
> Click **Finish**.
> Click **Return to Medication Room**.

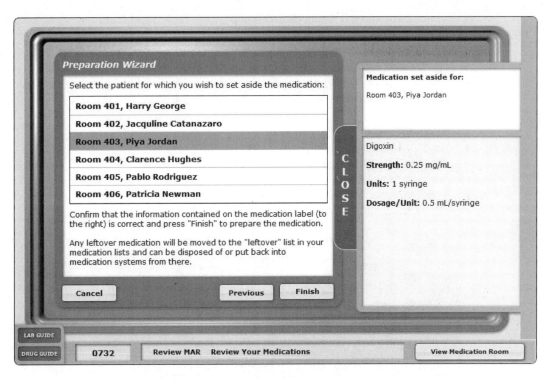

Follow this same basic process for the other medications due to be administered to Piya Jordan during this period of care. (*Hint:* Look in **IV Storage** and **Automated System**.)

PREPARATION WIZARD EXCEPTIONS

- Some medications in *Virtual Clinical Excursions—Medical-Surgical* are preprepared by the pharmacy (e.g., IV antibiotics) and taken to the patient room as a whole. This is common practice in most hospitals.
- Blood products are not administered by students through the *Virtual Clinical Excursions— Medical-Surgical* simulations because blood administration follows specific protocols not covered in this program.
- The *Virtual Clinical Excursions—Medical-Surgical* simulations do not allow for mixing more than one type of medication, such as regular and Lente insulins, in the same syringe. In the clinical setting, when multiple types of insulin are ordered for a patient, the regular insulin is drawn up first, followed by the longer-acting insulin. Insulin is always administered in a special unit-marked syringe.

Now return to Room 403 (click on **403** on the bottom tool bar) to administer Piya Jordan's medications.

At any time during the medication administration process, you can perform a further review of systems, take vital signs, check information contained within the chart, or verify patient identity and allergies. Inside Piya Jordan's room, click **Take Vital Signs**. (*Note:* These findings change over time to reflect the temporal changes you would find in a patient similar to Piya Jordan.)

When you have gathered all the data you need, click on **Patient Care** and then select **Medication Administration**. Any medications you prepared in the previous steps should be listed on the left side of your screen. Let's continue the administration process with the digoxin ordered for Piya Jordan. Click to highlight **Digoxin** in the list of medications. Next, click on the down arrow to the right of **Select** and choose **Administer** from the drop-down menu. This will activate the Administration Wizard. Complete the Wizard sequence as follows:

- Route: **IV**
- Method: **Direct Injection**
- Site: **Peripheral IV**
- Click **Administer to Patient** arrow.
- Would you like to document this administration in the MAR? **Yes**
- Click **Finish** arrow.

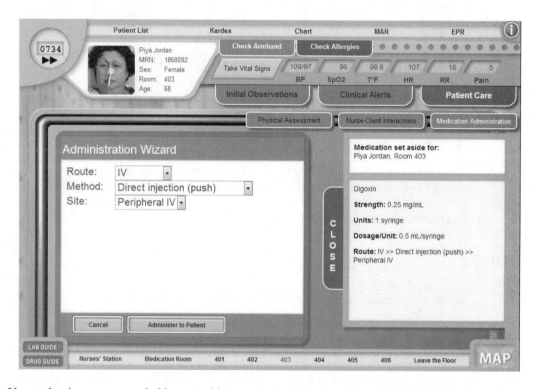

Your selections are recorded by a tracking system and evaluated on a Medication Scorecard stored under Preceptor's Evaluations. This scorecard can be viewed, printed, and given to your instructor. To access the Preceptor's Evaluations, click on **Leave the Floor**. When the Floor Menu appears, select **Look at Your Preceptor's Evaluation**. Then click on **Medication Scorecard** inside the box with Piya Jordan's name (see example on the following page).

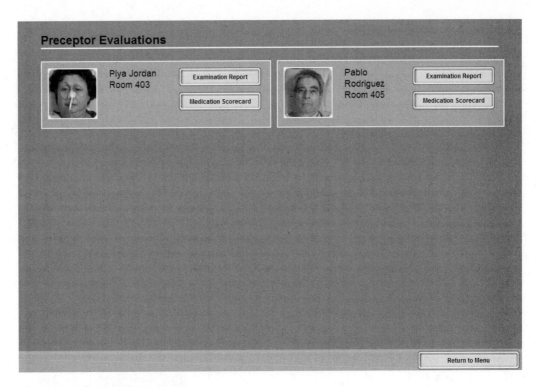

■ MEDICATION SCORECARD

- First, review Table A. Was digoxin given correctly? Did you give the other medications as ordered?
- Table B shows you which (if any) medications you gave incorrectly.
- Table C addresses the resources used for Piya Jordan. Did you access the patient's chart, MAR, EPR, or Kardex as needed to make safe medication administration decisions?
- Did you check the patient's armband to verify her identity? Did you check whether your patient had any known allergies to medications? Were vital signs taken?

When you have finished reviewing the scorecard, click **Return to Evaluations** and then **Return to Menu**.

■ **VITAL SIGNS**

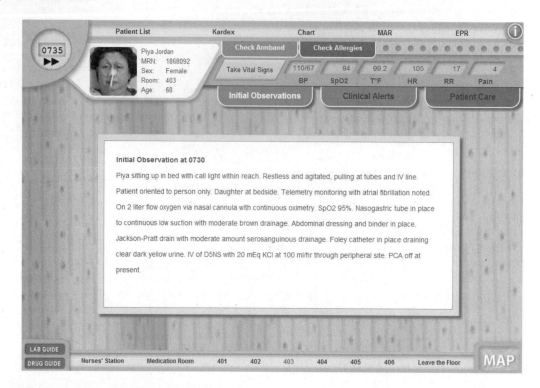

Vital signs, often considered the traditional "signs of life," include body temperature, heart rate, respiratory rate, blood pressure, oxygen saturation of the blood, and pain level.

Inside Piya Jordan's room, click **Take Vital Signs**. (*Note:* If you are following this detailed tour step by step, you will need to **Restart the Program** from the Floor Menu, sign in again for Period of Care 1, and navigate to Room 403.) Collect vital signs for this patient and record them below. Note the time at which you collected each of these data. (*Remember:* You can take vital signs at any time. The data change over time to reflect the temporal changes you would find in a patient similar to Piya Jordan.)

Vital Signs	Findings/Time
Blood pressure	
O$_2$ saturation	
Temperature	
Heart rate	
Respiratory rate	
Pain rating	

After you are done, click on the **EPR** icon located in the tool bar at the top of the screen. Your username and password are automatically provided. Click on **Login** to enter the EPR. To access Piya Jordan's records, click on the down arrow next to Patient and choose her room number, **403**. Select **Vital Signs** as the category. Next, in the empty time column on the far right, record the vital signs data you just collected in Piya Jordan's room. If you need help with this process, refer to the Electronic Patient Record (EPR) section of the Quick Tour. Now compare these findings with the data you collected earlier for this patient's vital signs. Use these earlier findings to establish a baseline for each of the vital signs.

    a.   Are any of the data you collected significantly different from the baseline for a particular vital sign?

        Circle One: Yes   No

    b.   If "Yes," which data are different?

■ **PHYSICAL ASSESSMENT**

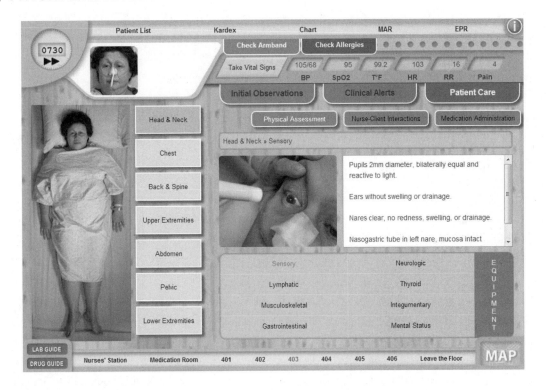

After you have finished examining the EPR for vital signs, click **Exit EPR** to return to Room 403. Click **Patient Care** and then **Physical Assessment**. Think about the information you received in the report at the beginning of this shift, as well as what you may have learned about this patient from the chart. Based on this, what area(s) of examination should you pay most attention to at this time? Is there any equipment you should be monitoring? Conduct a physical assessment of the body areas and systems that you consider priorities for Piya Jordan. For example, select **Head & Neck**; then click on and assess **Sensory** and **Lymphatic**. Complete any other assessment(s) you think are necessary at this time. In the following table, record the data you collected during this examination.

Area of Examination	Findings
Head & Neck Sensory	
Head & Neck Lymphatic	

After you have finished collecting these data, return to the EPR. Compare the data that were already in the record with those you just collected.

a. Are any of the data you collected significantly different from the baselines for this patient?

Circle One: Yes   No

b. If "Yes," which data are different?

■ NURSE-CLIENT INTERACTIONS

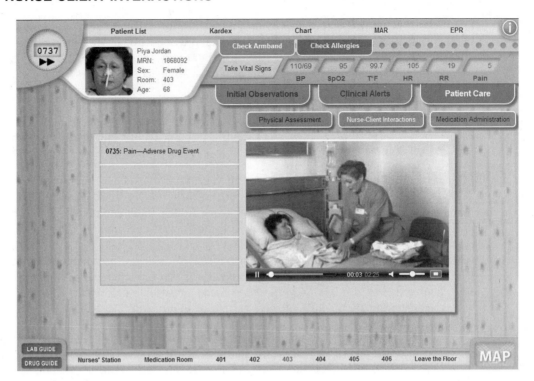

Click on **Patient Care** from inside Piya Jordan's room (403). Now click on **Nurse-Client Interactions** to access a short video titled **Pain—Adverse Drug Event**, which is available for viewing at or after 0735 (based on the virtual clock in the upper left corner of your screen; see *Note* below). To begin the video, click on the white arrow next to its title. You will observe a nurse communicating with Piya Jordan and her daughter. There are many variations of nursing practice, some exemplifying "best" practice and some not. Note whether the nurse in this interaction displays professional behavior and compassionate care. Are her words congruent with what is going on with the patient? Does this interaction "feel right" to you? If not, how would you handle this situation differently? Explain.

Note: If the video you wish to view is not listed, this means you have not yet reached the correct virtual time to view that video. Check the virtual clock; you may return to access the video once its designated time has occurred—as long as you do so within the same period of care. Or you can click on the fast-forward icon within the virtual clock to advance the time by 2-minute intervals. You will then need to click again on **Patient Care** and **Nurse-Client Interactions** to refresh the screen.

At least one Nurse-Client Interactions video is available during each period of care. Viewing these videos can help you learn more about what is occurring with a patient at a certain time and also prompt you to discern between nurse communications that are ideal and those that need improvement. Compassionate care and the ability to communicate clearly are essential components of delivering quality nursing care, and it is during your clinical time that you will begin to refine these skills.

■ COLLECTING AND EVALUATING DATA

Each of the activities you perform in the Patient Care environment generates a significant amount of assessment data. Remember that after you collect data, you can record your findings in the EPR. You can also review the EPR, patient's chart, videos, and MAR at any time. You will get plenty of practice collecting and then evaluating data in context of the patient's course.

Now, here's an important question for you:

> Did the previous sequence of exercises provide the most efficient way to assess Piya Jordan?

For example, you went to the patient's room to get vital signs, then back to the EPR to enter data and compare your findings with extant data. Next, you went back to the patient's room to do a physical examination, then again back to the EPR to enter and review data. If this back-and-forth process of data collection and recording seemed inefficient, remember the following:

- Plan all of your nursing activities to maximize efficiency, while at the same time optimizing the quality of patient care. (Think about what data you might need before performing certain tasks. For example, do you need to check a heart rate before administering a cardiac medication or check an IV site before starting an infusion?)

- You collect a tremendous amount of data when you work with a patient. Very few people can accurately remember all these data for more than a few minutes. Develop efficient assessment skills, and record data as soon as possible after collecting them.

- Assessment data are only the starting point for the nursing process.

Make a clear distinction between these first exercises and how you actually provide nursing care. These initial exercises were designed to involve you actively in the use of different software components. This workbook focuses on sensible practices for implementing the nursing process in ways that ensure the highest-quality care of patients.

Most important, remember that a human being changes through time, and that these changes include both the physical and psychosocial facets of a person as a living organism. Think about this for a moment. Some patients may change physically in a very short time (a patient with emerging myocardial infarction) or more slowly (a patient with a chronic illness). Patients' overall physical and psychosocial conditions may improve or deteriorate. They may have effective coping skills and familial support, or they may feel alone and full of despair. In fact, each individual is a complex mix of physical and psychosocial elements, and at least some of these elements usually change through time.

Thus it is crucial that you *DO NOT* think of the nursing process as a simple one-time, five-step procedure consisting of assessment, nursing diagnosis, planning, implementation, and evaluation. Rather, the nursing process should be utilized as a creative and systematic approach to delivering nursing care. Furthermore, because all living organisms are constantly changing, we must apply the nursing process over and over. Each time we follow the nursing process for an individual patient, we refine our understanding of that patient's physical and psychosocial conditions based on collection and analysis of many different types of data. *Virtual Clinical Excursions—Medical-Surgical* will help you develop both the creativity and the systematic approach needed to become a nurse who is equipped to deliver the highest-quality care to all patients.

REDUCING MEDICATION ERRORS

REDUCING MEDICATION ERRORS

Earlier in the detailed tour, you learned the basic steps of medication preparation and administration. The following simulations will allow you to practice those skills further—with an increased emphasis on reducing medication errors by using the Medication Scorecard to evaluate your work.

Sign in to work at Pacific View Regional Hospital for Period of Care 1. (*Note:* If you are already working with another patient or during another period of care, click on **Leave the Floor** and then **Restart the Program**; then sign in.)

From the Patient List, select Clarence Hughes. Then click on **Go to Nurses' Station**. Complete the following steps to prepare and administer medications to Clarence Hughes.

- Click on **Medication Room** on the tool bar at the bottom of your screen.
- Click on **MAR** and then on tab **404** to determine medications that have been ordered for Clarence Hughes. (*Note:* You may click on **Review MAR** at any time to verify the correct medication order. Always remember to check the patient name on the MAR to make sure you have the correct patient's record. You must click on the correct room number tab within the MAR.) Click on **Return to Medication Room** after reviewing the correct MAR.
- Click on **Unit Dosage** (or on the Unit Dosage cabinet); from the close-up view, click on drawer **404**.
- Select the medications you would like to administer. After each selection, click **Put Medication on Tray**. When you are finished selecting medications, click **Close Drawer** and then **View Medication Room**.
- Click on **Automated System** (or on the Automated System unit itself). Click **Login**.
- On the next screen, specify the correct patient and drawer location.
- Select the medication you would like to administer and click on **Put Medication on Tray**. Repeat this process if you wish to administer other medications from the Automated System.
- When you are finished, click **Close Drawer** and **View Medication Room**.
- From the Medication Room, click on **Preparation** (or on the preparation tray).
- From the list of medications on your tray, highlight the correct medication to administer and click **Prepare**.
- This activates the Preparation Wizard. Supply any requested information; then click **Next**.
- Now select the correct patient to receive this medication and click **Finish**.
- Repeat the previous three steps until all medications that you want to administer are prepared.
- You can click on **Review Your Medications** and then on **Return to Medication Room** when ready. Once you are back in the Medication Room, go directly to Clarence Hughes' room by clicking on **404** at bottom of screen.
- Inside the patient's room, administer the medication, utilizing the six rights of medication administration. After you have collected the appropriate assessment data and are ready for administration, click **Patient Care** and then **Medication Administration**. Verify that the correct patient and medication(s) appear in the left-hand window. Highlight the first medication you wish to administer; then click the down arrow next to Select. From the drop-down menu, select **Administer** and complete the Administration Wizard by providing any information requested. When the Wizard stops asking for information, click **Administer to Patient**. Specify **Yes** when asked whether this administration should be recorded in the MAR. Finally, click **Finish**.

■ SELF-EVALUATION

Now let's see how you did during your medication administration!

- Click on **Leave the Floor** at the bottom of your screen. From the Floor Menu, select **Look at Your Preceptor's Evaluation**. Then click **Medication Scorecard**.

The following exercises will help you identify medication errors, investigate possible reasons for these errors, and reduce or prevent medication errors in the future.

1. Start by examining Table A. These are the medications you should have given to Clarence Hughes during this period of care. If each of the medications in Table A has a ✓ by it, then you made no errors. Congratulations!

If any medication has an X by it, then you made one or more medication errors.

Compare Tables A and B to determine which of the following types of errors you made: Wrong Dose, Wrong Route/Method/Site, or Wrong Time. Follow these steps:
   a. Find medications in Table A that were given incorrectly.
   b. Now see if those same medications are in Table B, which shows what you actually administered to Clarence Hughes.
   c. Comparing Tables A and B, match the Strength, Dose, Route/Method/Site, and Time for each medication you administered incorrectly.
   d. Then, using the form below, list the medications given incorrectly and mark the errors you made for each medication.

Medication	Strength	Dosage	Route	Method	Site	Time
	❑	❑	❑	❑	❑	❑
	❑	❑	❑	❑	❑	❑
	❑	❑	❑	❑	❑	❑
	❑	❑	❑	❑	❑	❑

2. To help you reduce future medication errors, consider the following list of possible reasons for errors.

- Did not check drug against MAR for correct medication, correct dose, correct patient, correct route, correct time, correct documentation.
- Did not check drug dose against MAR three times.
- Did not open the unit dose package in the patient's room.
- Did not correctly identify the patient using two identifiers.
- Did not administer the drug on time.
- Did not verify patient allergies.
- Did not check the patient's current condition or vital sign parameters.
- Did not consider why the patient would be receiving this drug.
- Did not question why the drug was in the patient's drawer.
- Did not check the physician's order and/or check with the pharmacist when there was a question about the drug or dose.
- Did not verify that no adverse effects had occurred from a previous dose.

Based on the list of possibilities you just reviewed, determine how you made each error and record the reason in the form below:

Medication	Reason for Error

3. Look again at Table B. Are there medications listed that are not in Table A? If so, you gave a medication to Clarence Hughes that he should not have received. Complete the following exercises to help you understand how such an error might have been made.

   a. Perhaps you gave a medication that was on Clarence Hughes' MAR for this period of care, without recognizing that a change had occurred in the patient's condition, which should have caused you to reconsider. Review patient records as necessary and complete the following form:

Medication	Possible Reasons Not to Give This Medication

   b. Another possibility is that you gave Clarence Hughes a medication that should have been given at a different time. Check his MAR and complete the form below to determine whether you made a Wrong Time error:

Medication	Given to Clarence Hughes at What Time	Should Have Been Given at What Time

c. Maybe you gave another patient's medication to Clarence Hughes. In this case, you made a Wrong Patient error. Check the MARs of other patients and use the form below to determine whether you made this type of error:

Medication	Given to Clarence Hughes	Should Have Been Given to

4. The Medication Scorecard provides some other interesting sources of information. For example, if there is a medication selected for Clarence Hughes but it was not given to him, there will be an X by that medication in Table A, but it will not appear in Table B. In that case, you might have given this medication to some other patient, which is another type of Wrong Patient error. To investigate further, look at Table D, which lists the medications you gave to other patients. See whether you can find any medications ordered for Clarence Hughes that were given to another patient by mistake. However, before you make any decisions, be sure to cross-check the MAR for other patients because the same medication may have been ordered for multiple patients. Use the following form to record your findings:

Medication	Should Have Been Given to Clarence Hughes	Given by Mistake to

5. Now take some time to review the medication exercises you just completed. Use the form below to create an overall analysis of what you have learned. Once again, record each of the medication errors you made, including the type of each error. Then, for each error you made, indicate specifically what you would do differently to prevent this type of error from occurring again.

Medication	Type of Error	Error Prevention Tactic

Submit this form to your instructor if required as a graded assignment, or simply use these exercises to improve your understanding of medication errors and how to reduce them.

Name: _____   Date: _____

Pain

_____

Reading Assignment: Assessment and Care of Patients with Pain (Chapter 4)

Patients: Clarence Hughes, Room 404
Pablo Rodriguez, Room 405

Goal: To demonstrate understanding and appropriate application of pain management concepts.

Objectives:

1. Define the concept of *pain*.
2. Describe the source and type of pain experienced by a patient.
3. Perform a comprehensive pain assessment for a patient.
4. Identify variables that influence a patient's perception of pain.
5. Safely administer analgesic medications to a patient experiencing pain.
6. Plan appropriate nonpharmacologic measures that may be used to treat pain.

In this lesson you will evaluate the pain experience of two different patients from assessment to evaluation. Clarence Hughes is a 73-year-old male who is status post total knee arthroplasty. Pablo Rodriguez is a 71-year-old male admitted with advanced non-small cell lung carcinoma. Begin this activity by reviewing the general concepts presented in your textbook. Answer the following questions to solidify your understanding of pain.

Exercise 1

Writing Activity

5 minutes

1. Using the definitions of pain provided in the textbook, describe pain in your own words.

2. Match the type of pain with the correct description.

Type of Pain	Description
_____ Localized pain	a. Pain felt in an area distant from the site of painful stimuli
_____ Projected pain	b. Pain confined to the site of origin
_____ Radiating pain	c. Diffuse pain around the site of origin; is not well localized
_____ Referred pain	d. Pain felt along a specific nerve

3. When caring for a patient who is unable to verbalize pain, what indicators may be used to determine level of comfort?

Exercise 2

Virtual Hospital Activity

45 minutes

- Sign in to work at Pacific View Regional Hospital for Period of Care 1. (*Note:* If you are already in the virtual hospital from a previous exercise, click on **Leave the Floor** and then on **Restart the Program** to get to the sign-in window.)
- From the Patient List, select Clarence Hughes (Room 404) and then click on **Get Report**.

1. What data are provided in the report concerning this patient's most recent pain assessment?

Now review Clarence Hughes' medical history.

- Click on **Go to Nurses' Station**.
- Click on **Chart**.
- Click on **404**.
- Click on **History and Physical** and review.

2. Why has Clarence Hughes been admitted to the hospital?

Now complete your own pain assessment on Clarence Hughes.

- Click on **Return to Nurses' Station**.
- Click on **404** at the bottom of the screen.
- Click on **Take Vital Signs**.

3. How does Clarence Hughes rate his pain at this time?

- Click on **Patient Care** and then on **Nurse-Client Interactions**.
- Select and view the video titled **0730: Assessment/Perception of Care** (*Note:* Check the virtual clock to see whether enough time has elapsed. You can use the fast-forward feature to advance the time by 2-minute intervals if the video is not yet available. Click again on **Patient Care** and on **Nurse-Client Interactions** to refresh the screen.)

4. How does Clarence Hughes describe his pain? Describe his nonverbal communication. Do his nonverbal cues correlate with his complaint of pain?

5. The nurse asks Clarence Hughes whether she may perform an assessment before medicating him for pain. Is this appropriate? Why or why not?

6. What elements are missing from the discussion between Clarence Hughes and the nurse?

7. Considering the physiologic source of Clarence Hughes' pain, which descriptive terms would most likely be reported? Select all that apply.

_____ Poorly localized

_____ Sharp

_____ Shooting

_____ Burning

_____ Aching

_____ Dull

_____ Cramping

- Use the fast-forward feature to advance the virtual clock to 0745.
- Click on **Patient Care** and then on **Physical Assessment**.
- Perform a focused assessment by clicking on the body system categories (yellow buttons) and body system subcategories (green buttons).

8. Document the findings of your physical assessment below.

- Click on **EPR**. Click on **Login**.
- Select **404** from the Patient drop-down menu and **Vital Signs** from the Category drop-down menu.

9. Describe the characteristics of Clarence Hughes' pain over the last 24 hours (Tuesday at 0700 through Wednesday at 0715). Select all that apply.

_____   Ache

_____   Burning

_____   Constant

_____   Dull

_____   Electric

_____   External

_____   Intermittent

_____   Internal

_____   Radiating

_____   Sharp

_____   Shooting

- Click on **Return to Nurses' Station**.
- Click on **Chart** and then on **404**.
- Click on **Kardex** and then on tab **404**.

10. What is the stated outcome related to comfort for Clarence Hughes? Is this a measurable outcome? How might you improve on the writing of the outcome?

- Click on **Return to Nurses' Station**.
- Click on **Chart** and then on **404**.
- Click on **Expired MARs**.

11. Record the PRN pain medication administration times for Tuesday.

- Click on **Return to Nurses' Station**.
- Click on **EPR** and then on **Login**.
- Select **404** from the Patient drop-down menu and **Vital Signs** from the Category menu.

12. Review the pain ratings and characteristics documented for Tuesday, beginning at 0815. Based on the stated outcome related to comfort, was the pain medication effective? Give a rationale for your answer.

13. Review the follow-up pain assessments documented after each of the pain medication administrations on Tuesday. Was the patient's pain assessed appropriately following the administration of each analgesic? Explain your answer.

14. Is the ordered analgesic medication appropriate for this type of pain? If not, what would you suggest? Are there any nonpharmacologic interventions that might be helpful for Clarence Hughes? Explain your answer.

15. What assessments should the nurse complete before administering oxycodone with acetaminophen?

16. For what common side effects related to opioid use should the nurse monitor? (*Hint:* If you need help, return to the Nurses' Station and click on the **Drug Guide** on the counter.)

- Click on **Return to Room 404**.
- Click on **Chart** and then on **404**.
- Click on the **Nurse's Notes** tab and review the record.

17. According to the note for Wednesday at 0715, which of the side effects identified in question 16 is Clarence Hughes experiencing? What should the nurse do to treat and/or prevent this side effect?

Clarence Hughes received his last dose of pain medication at 0200. It is now appropriate to administer another dose. Prepare to administer a dose of analgesic to him by completing the following steps:

- Click on **Return to Nurses' Station**.
- Click on **Medication Room** on the bottom of your screen.
- Click on **Automated System**.
- Click on **Login**.
- Select Clarence Hughes from box 1 and Automated System Drawer (G-O) from box 2.
- Click on **Open Drawer** and review the list of available medications. (*Note:* You may click on **Review MAR** at any time to verify medication orders. Click on the correct room number within the MAR. Remember to look at the patient name on the MAR to make sure you have the correct patient's record. Click on **Return to Medication Room** after reviewing the correct MAR.)

- From the Open Drawer view, select the correct medication to administer. Click on **Put Medication on Tray** and then on **Close System Drawer**.
- Click on **View Medication Room**.
- Click on **Preparation**. On the next screen, click on the name of the medication to select it.
- Click on **Prepare Medication**, fill in any requested data in the Preparation Wizard, and then click on **Next**.
- Select the correct patient and click on **Finish**.
- You can click on **Review Your Medications** and then on **Return to Medication Room** when ready.
- Click on **404** at the bottom of your screen.
- Administer the medication utilizing the six rights of medication administration. After you have collected the appropriate assessment data and are ready to administer the medication, click on **Patient Care** and then on **Medication Administration**.
- Verify that the correct patient and medication(s) appear in the left-hand window. Click on the down arrow next to Select.
- From the drop-down menu, select **Administer** and complete the Administration Wizard by providing any information requested.
- When the Wizard stops asking for information, click on **Administer to Patient**. Specify **Yes** when asked whether this administration should be recorded in the MAR.
- Finally, click on **Finish**.

Now let's see how you did!

- Click on **Leave the Floor** at the bottom of your screen.
- From the Floor Menu, click on **Look at Your Preceptor's Evaluation**.
- Click on **Medication Scorecard**.

18. Disregard the report for the routine scheduled medications, and instead note below whether or not you correctly administered the analgesic medication. If not, why do you think you were incorrect in administering this drug? According to Table C in this scorecard, what are the appropriate resources that should be used before administering this medication? Did you utilize them correctly?

19. The nurse caring for Clarence Hughes should be aware that his tolerance to the drowsiness caused by

opioid analgesics will be reached in _____.

Exercise 3

Virtual Hospital Activity

45 minutes

- Sign in to work at Pacific View Regional Hospital for Period of Care 1. (*Note:* If you are already in the virtual hospital from a previous exercise, click on **Leave the Floor** and then on **Restart the Program** to get to the sign-in window.)
- From the Patient List, select Pablo Rodriguez (Room 405).
- Click on **Get Report**.

1. What information is provided in the report concerning Pablo Rodriguez's most recent pain assessment?

- Click on **Go to Nurses' Station**.
- Click on **Chart**.
- Click on **405**.
- Click on **History and Physical** and review.

2. What is Pablo Rodriguez's medical diagnosis?

Now let's complete your own pain assessment on Pablo Rodriguez.

- Click on **Return to Nurses' Station**.
- Click on **405** at the bottom of your screen.
- Click on **Take Vital Signs**.

3. How does Pablo Rodriguez rate his pain at the present time?

- Click on **Patient Care** and then on **Physical Assessment**.
- Perform a focused assessment by clicking on the body system categories (yellow buttons) and body system subcategories (green buttons).

4. Document the findings of your physical assessment below.

- Click on **Chart** and then on **405**.
- Click on **Nursing Admission**. Scroll down to the Comfort section.

5. What are the aggravating and alleviating factors related to Pablo Rodriguez's pain?

- Click on **Return to Room 405**.
- Click on **Patient Care** and then on **Nurse-Client Interactions**.
- Select and view the video titled **0730: Symptom Management**. (*Note:* Check the virtual clock to see whether enough time has elapsed. You can use the fast-forward feature to advance the time by 2-minute intervals if the video is not yet available. Then click again on **Patient Care** and on **Nurse-Client Interactions** to refresh the screen.)

6. Discuss the nurse's evaluation of Pablo Rodriguez's understanding and use of the PCA pump. Do you think the nurse's actions are therapeutic? If not, what other approaches would you suggest?

7. What nursing assessments and interventions are appropriate for patients receiving IV morphine sulfate? (*Hint:* For help, click on the **Drug** icon in the lower left corner of the screen.)

- Click on **EPR**.
- Click on **Login**.
- Select **405** from the Patient drop-down menu and **Vital Signs** from the Category drop-down menu.

8. Describe the characteristics of Pablo Rodriquez's pain during his stay. Select all that apply.

_____ Ache

_____ Burning

_____ Constant

_____ Dull

_____ Electric

_____ External

_____ Intermittent

_____ Internal

_____ Radiating

_____ Sharp

_____ Shooting

- Now click on **Return to Room 405**.
- Click on **Kardex**.
- Click on **405** and review the record for Pablo Rodriguez.

9. What is the stated outcome related to comfort for Pablo Rodriguez? Is this a measurable outcome? How might you improve on the writing of the outcome?

- Now click on **Return to Room 405**.
- Click on **Chart** and then on **405**.
- Click on **Expired MARs**.

10. Record the pain medications, including dosage, route, and time received.

- Click on **Return to Room 405**.
- Click on **EPR** and then on **Login**.

11. Was the patient's pain assessed appropriately following each administration of analgesic? Explain your answer.

12. What type of pain is Pablo Rodriguez experiencing? What is the physiologic source for this pain? Explain your answer.

13. Is the ordered analgesic medication appropriate for this type of pain? If not, what would you suggest? Are there any nonpharmacologic interventions that might be helpful for Pablo Rodriguez? Explain your answer.

- Click on **Return to Room 405**.
- Click on **Patient Care** and then on **Nurse-Client Interactions**.
- Select and view the video titled **0735: Patient Perceptions**. (*Note:* Check the virtual clock to see whether enough time has elapsed. You can use the fast-forward feature to advance the time by 2-minute intervals if the video is not yet available. Then click again on **Patient Care** and on **Nurse-Client Interactions** to refresh the screen.)

14. What cultural influences are affecting this patient's perception and management of pain?

End-of-Life Care

Reading Assignment: End-of-Life Care Concepts (Chapter 7)

Patient: Pablo Rodriguez, Room 405

Goal: To demonstrate understanding and appropriate application of end-of-life concepts related to health care.

Objectives:

1. Identify appropriate application of palliative care concepts for a patient with a terminal illness.
2. Assess and identify common symptoms of distress present in a terminally ill patient.
3. Choose interventions appropriate to relieve symptoms of distress in a terminally ill patient.
4. Describe appropriate communication techniques to use when dealing with a terminally ill patient and family.

In this lesson you will describe, plan, and evaluate the care of a patient with a terminal illness that is no longer responding to therapy. Pablo Rodriguez is a 71-year-old male suffering from advanced non-small cell lung carcinoma diagnosed 1 year ago.

Exercise 1

Virtual Hospital Activity

30 minutes

- Sign in to work at Pacific View Regional Hospital for Period of Care 3. (*Note:* If you are already in the virtual hospital from a previous exercise, click on **Leave the Floor** and then on **Restart the Program** to get to the sign-in window.)
- From the Patient List, select Pablo Rodriguez (Room 405).
- Click on **Go to Nurses' Station**.
- Click on **Chart** and then on **405**.
- Click on **Emergency Department** and review this record.

1. Why was Pablo Rodriguez admitted to the hospital?

2. What are Pablo Rodriguez's primary and secondary diagnoses?

• Click on **Admissions**.

3. Review the information concerning advance directives in the chart. What is Pablo Rodriguez's current status with regard to this document?

4. Which are guidelines included in the Patient Self-Determination Act of 1991? Select all that apply.

_____ Patients admitted to health care agencies must be asked if they have executed an advance directive (AD).

_____ Physician offices must initiate AD inquiries with patients planning to be admitted to a clinical facility.

_____ For those patients who have not executed an AD, health care agencies must provide them with information regarding the value of ADs.

_____ For those patients who have not executed an AD, health care agencies must provide them with the opportunity to complete the state-required forms.

_____ The patient must have written permission from the attending physician to enact a presented AD.

_____ ADs require an attorney for completion.

_____ AD laws vary by state.

5. To retain health care decision-making responsibilities, which criteria must be met by the patient? Select all that apply.

_____ The patient must be alert and oriented x 4.

_____ The patient must be able to receive information provided by health care providers.

_____ The patient must be able to communicate treatment choices.

_____ The patient must have the cognitive ability to evaluate treatment options.

• Click on **Return to Nurses' Station**.
• Click on **Kardex**.
• Click on **405**.

6. What is Pablo Rodriguez's code status? Is this appropriate based on the reason for this admission? Explain.

• Click on **Return to Nurses' Station**.
• Click on **405** at the bottom of your screen.
• Click on **Patient Care** and then on **Nurse-Client Interactions**.
• Select and view the video titled **1530: Decision—End-of-Life Care**. (*Note:* Check the virtual clock to see whether enough time has elapsed. You can use the fast-forward feature to advance the time by 2-minute intervals if the video is not yet available. Then click again on **Patient Care** and on **Nurse-Client Interactions** to refresh the screen.)

7. What is Pablo Rodriguez telling the nurse?

8. What therapeutic communication techniques is the nurse using? Are they effective? What other technique(s) might have been used?

9. What would you do if Pablo Rodriguez asked you to administer a lethal dose of morphine to "stop my pain and help me die with dignity"? What legal term would apply to this request?

10. How do passive euthanasia and active euthanasia differ?

Exercise 2

Virtual Hospital Activity

45 minutes

- Sign in to work at Pacific View Regional Hospital for Period of Care 1. (*Note:* If you are already in the virtual hospital from a previous exercise, click on **Leave the Floor** and then on **Restart the Program** to get to the sign-in window.)
- From the Patient List, select Pablo Rodriguez (Room 405).
- Click on **Go to Nurses' Station**.
- Click on **405** at the bottom of your screen.
- Read the Initial Observations.

1. What physical symptom of distress is Pablo Rodriguez displaying?

2. Identify interventions you would use to alleviate Pablo Rodriguez's symptoms. Provide rationales for your interventions. (*Hint:* You may need to go to the patient's chart to review physician orders and/or use the Drug Guide to provide rationales.)

- Click on **EPR**.
- Click on **Login**.
- Choose **405** from the Patient drop-down menu and **Vital Signs** from the Category drop-down menu.
- Find the vital signs assessment documented at 0700.

3. Describe Pablo Rodriguez's pain assessment.

- Click on **Return to Room 405**.
- Click on **MAR** and then on tab **405**.

4. What pharmacologic interventions would be appropriate to relieve this pain? What nonpharmacologic interventions would you suggest?

Now let's check the patient's current vital signs.

- Click on **Return to Room 405**.
- Click on **Take Vital Signs**.

5. Based on the EPR data and Pablo Rodriguez's current pain rating, is the morphine providing effective relief? Explain.

- Click on **Patient Care** and then on **Physical Assessment**.
- Click on **Abdomen** (yellow button).
- Click on **Gastrointestinal** (green button).

6. Document your assessment findings below. What is this significance of these findings? How do they relate to Pablo Rodriguez's diagnosis and/or treatment?

- Click on **MAR** and then on tab **405**.

7. What pharmacologic and nonpharmacologic interventions would you implement to prevent potential complications related to the above findings?

- Click on **Return to Room 405**.
- Click on **Patient Care** and then on **Nurse-Client Interactions**.
- Select and view the video titled **0730: Symptom Management**. (*Note:* Check the virtual clock to see whether enough time has elapsed. You can use the fast-forward feature to advance the time by 2-minute intervals if the video is not yet available. Then click again on **Patient Care** and on **Nurse-Client Interactions** to refresh the screen.)

8. Now that his pain has been controlled, what two physical symptoms of distress does Pablo Rodriguez complain of? For each of his symptoms, identify interventions you could use to relieve these discomforts.

- Select and view the video titled **0735: Patient Perceptions**. (*Note:* Check the virtual clock to see whether enough time has elapsed. You can use the fast-forward feature to advance the time by 2-minute intervals if the video is not yet available. Then click again on **Patient Care** and on **Nurse-Client Interactions** to refresh the screen.)

9. Describe Pablo Rodriguez's emotional distress as displayed in this video.

10. What nursing interventions would be appropriate to help Pablo Rodriguez cope?

11. Describe the nurse's role in end-of-life care. How does this compare with the care being provided for Pablo Rodriguez? Explain.

Fluid Imbalance

Reading Assignment: Assessment and Care of Patients with Problems of Fluid and
Electrolyte Balance (Chapter 11)

Patients: Piya Jordan, Room 403
Patricia Newman, Room 406

Goal: To utilize the nursing process to competently care for patients with fluid imbalances.

Objectives:

1. Identify normal physiologic influences on fluid and electrolyte balance.
2. Compare and contrast the pathophysiology related to dehydration and overhydration.
3. Utilize laboratory data and clinical manifestations to assess fluid balance and imbalance.
4. Describe collaborative management strategies used to maintain and/or restore fluid balance.
5. Critically analyze differences in the fluid balance assessment findings of two patients.
6. Develop an appropriate plan of care for patients displaying fluid imbalances.

In this lesson you will assess, plan, and implement care for two patients with similar but differing fluid imbalances. Piya Jordan is a 68-year-old female admitted with nausea and vomiting for several days following weeks of poor appetite and increasing weakness. Patricia Newman is a 61-year-old female admitted with dyspnea at rest, cough, and fever. You will begin this lesson by reviewing the general concepts of fluid homeostasis as presented in your textbook. Answer the following questions to cement your understanding of the normal physiologic concepts related to fluid balance.

Exercise 1

Writing Activity

30 minutes

1. Describe the function of water in the body.

2. Identify the two main water (fluid) compartments in the body and describe the composition of each.

3. Describe the pathophysiology for dehydration and identify key clinical manifestations.

4. Describe the pathophysiology of fluid volume overload and identify key clinical manifestations.

5. Match each term related to fluid volume regulation with its corresponding definition.

Term	**Definition**
_____ Hydrostatic pressure	a. The free movement of particles (solute) across a permeable membrane from an area of higher concentration to an area of lower concentration
_____ Filtration	
	b. The movement of fluid through a cell or blood vessel membrane because of hydrostatic pressure differences on both sides of the membrane
_____ Diffusion	
_____ Osmolarity	c. The movement of water only through a selectively permeable (semipermeable) membrane
_____ Aldosterone	
_____ Hypotonic	d. The pressing of water molecules against confining walls
_____ Osmosis	e. The number of milliosmoles in a kilogram of solution
_____ Antidiuretic hormone (ADH)	f. The number of milliosmoles in a liter of solution
	g. The particles dissolved or suspended in water
_____ Isotonic	
_____ Osmolality	h. A fluid with a solute concentration equal to the osmolarity of normal body fluids or normal saline, about 300 mOsm/L
_____ Solute	i. Diffusion across a cell membrane that requires the assistance of a membrane-altering system
_____ Facilitated diffusion	
	j. A hormone secreted by the adrenal cortex whenever sodium levels in the extracellular fluid (ECF) are decreased
_____ Hypertonic	
	k. A fluid with an osmolarity greater than 300 mOsm/L
	l. A fluid with an osmolarity less than that of normal body fluids (less than 270 mOsm/L)
	m. A hormone produced in the brain that is stored in and released from the posterior pituitary gland in response to changes in blood osmolarity

Exercise 2

Virtual Hospital Activity

20 minutes

- Sign in to work at Pacific View Regional Hospital for Period of Care 1. (*Note:* If you are already in the virtual hospital from a previous exercise, click on **Leave the Floor** and then on **Restart the Program** to get to the sign-in window.)
- From the Patient List, select Piya Jordan (Room 403).
- Click on **Go to Nurses' Station**.
- Click on **Chart** and then on **403**.
- Click on **Emergency Department** and review the record.

1. Record findings below that support the diagnosis of dehydration.

- Click on **Nursing Admission**.

2. Are there any additional findings noted on this document that support the diagnosis of dehydration? If so, list them below.

- Click on **Laboratory Reports**.

3. Record all pertinent results for Monday at 2200 below and describe the significance of each result in relation to the diagnosis of dehydration.

• Click on **History and Physical.**

4. Based on your review of Piya Jordan's History and Physical, what were the contributing factors leading to her dehydration?

• Click on **Physician's Orders**.

5. Identify orders on Monday at 2115 that represent appropriate management strategies for the treatment of dehydration and write your findings below.

Exercise 3

Virtual Hospital Activity

45 minutes

Now you will answer similar questions related to fluid balance for another patient and compare your findings.

• Sign in to work at Pacific View Regional Hospital for Period of Care 1. (*Note:* If you are already in the virtual hospital from a previous exercise, click on **Leave the Floor** and then on **Restart the Program** to get to the sign-in window.)
• From the Patient List, select Patricia Newman (Room 406).
• Click on **Go to Nurses' Station**.
• Click on **Chart** and then on **406**.
• Click on **Emergency Department** and review this record.

1. Identify assessment findings for Patricia Newman related to fluid balance and record them below. How do these findings differ from those for Piya Jordan? Are there any similarities?

- Click on **Nursing Admission**.

2. Are there any additional findings noted on this document related to fluid balance and/or imbalance? If so, list them below. How do they compare with findings for Piya Jordan?

- Click on **Laboratory Results**.

3. Record all pertinent results from Tuesday at 2300 and Wednesday at 0500 below and describe the significance of each result in relation to fluid balance. Describe any differences between these findings and Piya Jordan's findings.

4. Based on your findings, does Patricia Newman have a fluid imbalance? If so, what type?

5. What are the contributing factors for this patient's potential or actual fluid imbalance?

- Click on **History and Physical**.

6. What coexisting illness might have an impact on the selection and rate of IV fluid therapy?

7. Develop a plan of care for the patient with dehydration.

Nursing diagnosis

Assessment parameters

Diet therapy

Drug therapy

8. Develop a plan of care for the patient with fluid volume overload.

Nursing diagnosis

Assessment parameters

Diet therapy

Drug therapy

Electrolyte Imbalances, Part 1

_____

Reading Assignment: Assessment and Care of Patients with Problems of Fluid and
                          Electrolyte Balance (Chapter 11)

Patients: Piya Jordan, Room 403
               Patricia Newman, Room 406

Goal: To utilize the nursing process to competently care for patients with electrolyte imbalances.

Objectives:

  1. Describe normal physiologic influences on electrolyte balance.
  2. Identify specific etiologic factors related to hypokalemia for assigned patients.
  3. Research potential drug interactions related to hypokalemia for assigned patients.
  4. Assess patients for clinical manifestations related to hypo- and hyperkalemia.
  5. Utilize the nursing process to correctly administer IV potassium chloride per physician orders.

In this lesson you will assess, plan, and implement care for two patients with hypokalemia. Piya Jordan is a
68-year-old female admitted with nausea and vomiting for several days following weeks of poor appetite
and increasing weakness. Patricia Newman is a 61-year-old female admitted with pneumonia and a 12-year
history of emphysema. You will begin this lesson by reviewing the general functions of electrolytes within
the body as presented in your textbook. Answer the following questions to cement your understanding of
the normal physiologic concepts related to potassium balance.

Exercise 1

Writing Activity

10 minutes

  1. Describe the general function of electrolytes.

2. Match each term with its corresponding definition.

Term	Definition
_____ Anion	a. A negatively charged ion
_____ Cation	b. A substance in body fluids that carries an electrical charge; an electrolyte
_____ Ion	c. A positively charged ion

3. Match each condition with its potential corresponding potassium alteration. *(Hint:* See Table 11-1 in your textbook.)

Condition	Potential Potassium Alteration
_____ Fluid overload	a. Hypokalemia
_____ Alkalosis	b. Hyperkalemia
_____ Dehydration	
_____ Hyperaldosteronism	
_____ Kidney disease	

4. Identify the specific functions of potassium within the body. *(Hint:* See Chapter 11 in your textbook.)

5. Describe the physiologic influences on potassium balance.

Exercise 2

Virtual Hospital Activity

45 minutes

- Sign in to work at Pacific View Regional Hospital for Period of Care 1. (*Note:* If you are already in the virtual hospital from a previous exercise, click on **Leave the Floor** and then on **Restart the Program** to get to the sign-in window.)
- From the Patient List, select Piya Jordan (Room 403).
- Click on **Go to Nurses' Station.**
- Click on **Chart** and then on **403**.
- Click on **Laboratory Reports**.

1. What was Piya Jordan's initial potassium level on Monday at 2200?

2. When considering Piya Jordan's age, which is a therapeutic serum potassium level?
   a. 2.5 to 4.5 mEq/dL
   b. 3.5 to 5.0 mEq/L
   c. 4.0 to 6.0 mEq/L
   d. 4.0 to 6.5 mEq/L

- Click on **Emergency Department** and review this record.

3. What would be the most likely cause for hypokalemia in this patient? (*Hint:* See Table 11-7 in your textbook.)

- Click on **Physician's Orders**. Scroll down and review the orders for Monday at 2200.

4. What did the physician order to treat this electrolyte imbalance? Is this appropriate? Is the dilution and rate safe to administer? (*Hint:* See Chapter 11 in your textbook.)

- Click on **Laboratory Reports**.

5. What was Piya Jordan's potassium level for Tuesday at 0630? Was the physician's order for potassium replacement effective? Is there any other treatment ordered that would be a cause for concern?

6. When administering potassium chloride intravenously, what guidelines for the rate of administration should be observed?

- Click on **Return to Nurses' Station**.
- Click on **403** at the bottom of your screen.
- Click on **Patient Care** and then on **Physical Assessment**.
- Complete a physical assessment of Piya Jordan by clicking on the body categories (yellow buttons) and body subcategories (green buttons).
- Click on **Take Vital Signs**.

7. Specifically looking for clinical manifestations of hypokalemia, document your findings below for each area assessed.

Respiratory

Musculoskeletal

Cardiovascular

Neurologic

Intestinal

• Click on **Chart** and then on **403**. Then click on **Laboratory Reports**.

8. What was the potassium level that was drawn on Wednesday at 0630?

9. Explain the etiology for this recurrence of hypokalemia.

- Click on **Physician's Orders**.

10. What did the physician order in response to today's potassium level?

Prepare to administer this ordered dose of potassium chloride to Piya Jordan by completing the following steps.

- Click on **Return to Room 403**.
- Click on **Medication Room** on the bottom of your screen.
- Click on **IV Storage** near the top of your screen.
- Click on the bin labeled **Small Volume** and review the list of available medications. (*Note:* You may click on **Review MAR** at any time to verify correct medication order. Remember to click on the correct tab and to look at the patient name on the MAR to make sure you have the correct patient's record. Click on **Return to Medication Room** after reviewing the correct MAR.)
- From the list of medications in the bin, select **potassium chloride**.
- Click on **Put Medication on Tray** and then on **Close Bin**.
- Click on **View Medication Room**.
- Click on **Preparation**. Select the correct medication to administer; then click on **Prepare Medication**.
- Wait for instructions or questions from the Preparation Wizard. Then click on **Next**.
- Choose the correct patient to administer this medication to. Click on **Finish**.
- You can click on **Review Your Medications** and then on **Return to Medication Room** when ready. From the Medication Room, go directly to Piya Jordan's room by clicking on **403** at the bottom of your screen.

Before you administer IV medications, the patient's IV site must be assessed.

- Click on **Patient Care** and then on **Physical Assessment**.
- Click on **Upper Extremities**.
- Select **Integumentary** from the system subcategories.

11. Document the findings of your IV site assessment below. Is it appropriate to administer the IV potassium at this time?

- After you have collected the appropriate assessment data and are ready for administration, click on **Medication Administration**. (*Note:* If you are not still in the Patient Care screen, you will need to first click on **Patient Care** and then on **Medication Administration**.)
- On the left side of the window that appears, select the correct patient name and room number. If you prepared the patient's medication properly, the name of the medication will appear in the middle window.
- Click on the name of the medication you wish to administer. Then click **Administer** (near the bottom of the window).
- Complete the Administration Wizard and click **Administer to Patient** when done.
- Check **Yes** when asked whether this drug administration should be documented on the MAR and then click on **Finish**.
- Now click on **MAR** at the top of your screen.

12. What are Piya Jordan's scheduled morning medications? What medication would you question giving her, and for what reason? (*Hint:* See Chapter 11 in your textbook.)

13. Piya Jordan complains of pain at the IV site while the potassium is infusing. What interventions are appropriate at this time?

14. When considering pain at the site of the IV infusion, which manifestations are consistent with extravasation? Select all that apply.

_____ Pain

_____ Warmth

_____ Cool skin at site

_____ Absence of blood return

_____ Swelling

_____ Red streaking of skin over vein

Now let's see how you did!

- Click on **Leave the Floor** at the bottom of your screen. From the Floor Menu, select **Look at Your Preceptor's Evaluation**. Then click on **Medication Scorecard**.

15. Disregard the report for the routine scheduled medications, and instead note below whether or not you correctly administered the potassium chloride. If not, why do you think you were incorrect in administering this drug? According to Table C in this scorecard, what are the appropriate resources that should be used and important assessments that should be completed before administering this medication? Did you utilize and perform them correctly?

Exercise 3

Virtual Hospital Activity

30 minutes

- Sign in to work at Pacific View Regional Hospital for Period of Care 1. (*Note:* If you are still in the virtual hospital from a previous exercise, click on **Leave the Floor** and then on **Restart the Program** to get to the sign-in window.)
- From the Patient List, select Patricia Newman (Room 406).
- Click on **Go to Nurses' Station**.
- Click on **Chart** and then on **406**.
- Click on **Laboratory Reports**.

1. What was Patricia Newman's initial potassium level this morning?

- Click on **History and Physical**.

2. What would be the most likely cause for hypokalemia in this patient?

- Click on **Physician's Orders**.

3. What did the physician order on Wednesday at 0730 to treat this electrolyte imbalance?

4. What is missing from this order?

5. Where could you verify this missing information?

6. What is the difference between the treatment of hypokalemia for Piya Jordan and that for Patricia Newman? Provide a rationale for the difference.

7. Look again at the physician's orders. Is there an order for any follow-up lab work? What is the nurse's responsibility in regard to follow-up lab work, and how would you handle this situation?

8. When planning Patricia Newman's dietary intake, which selection is considered the best source of potassium?
   a. Salmon
   b. Eggs
   c. Bread
   d. Oatmeal

• Click on **Return to Nurses' Station**.
• Click on **406** at the bottom of your screen.
• Click on **Patient Care** and then on **Nurse-Client Interactions**.
• Select and view the video titled **0740: Evaluation—Response to Care**. (*Note:* Check the virtual clock to see whether enough time has elapsed. You can use the fast-forward feature to advance the time by 2-minute intervals if the video is not yet available. Then click again on **Patient Care** and on **Nurse-Client Interactions** to refresh the screen.)

9. Although Patricia Newman is happy that her chest does not hurt like it did, what does she verbalize as a concern?

10. How does the nurse respond to this expressed concern? Is it an adequate response?

11. For what clinical manifestations of hyperkalemia would you monitor Patricia Newman during her IV potassium therapy? (*Hint:* Consult the Drug Guide provided by clicking on the **Drug** icon in the lower left corner of your screen.)

Electrolyte Imbalances, Part 2

Reading Assignment: Assessment and Care of Patients with Problems of Fluid and Electrolyte Balance (Chapter 11)

Patient: Pablo Rodriguez, Room 405

Goal: To utilize the nursing process to competently care for patients with electrolyte imbalances.

Objectives:

1. Describe the pathophysiologic basis of electrolyte imbalances noted on a specific patient.
2. Identify specific etiologic factor(s) related to hypercalcemia, hyponatremia, and hypophosphatemia in the assigned patient.
3. Assess the assigned patient for clinical manifestations related to sodium, calcium, and phosphorus imbalances.
4. Describe appropriate nursing interventions to use when caring for a patient with hypercalcemia, hyponatremia, and hypophosphatemia.
5. Evaluate the effectiveness of medication prescribed to treat electrolyte imbalances.

In this lesson you will assess, plan, and implement care for a patient with several electrolyte imbalances. Pablo Rodriguez is a 71-year-old male who is admitted with nausea and vomiting for several days. He has a 1-year history of non-small cell lung carcinoma. You will begin this lesson by reviewing the general functions of specific electrolytes within the body as presented in your textbook. Answer the following questions to cement your understanding of the normal physiologic concepts related to phosphorus, sodium, chloride, and calcium balance.

Exercise 1

Writing Activity

20 minutes

1. Provide the following information for calcium.

   Normal level

   Functions

   Major location

   Mechanism(s) of electrolyte homeostasis

2. Provide the following information for phosphorous.

   Normal level

   Functions

   Major location

   Mechanism(s) of electrolyte homeostasis

3. Provide the following information for sodium.

Normal level

Functions

Major location

Mechanism(s) of electrolyte homeostasis

4. Provide the following information for chloride.

Normal level

Functions

Major location

Mechanism(s) of electrolyte homeostasis

Exercise 2

Virtual Hospital Activity

45 minutes

- Sign in to work at Pacific View Regional Hospital for Period of Care 1. (*Note:* If you are already in the virtual hospital from a previous exercise, click on **Leave the Floor** and then on **Restart the Program** to get to the sign-in window.)
- From the Patient List, select Pablo Rodriguez (Room 405).
- Click on **Go to Nurses' Station**.
- Click on **Chart** and then on **405**.
- Click on **Laboratory Reports**.

1. Record Pablo Rodriguez's serum chemistry results for Tuesday at 2000 and Wednesday at 0730, focusing on the areas listed below. Identify any abnormal values by marking as H (for high) or L (for low).

Sodium

Potassium

Chloride

Calcium

Phosphorus

Magnesium

- Click on **History and Physical** and review this record.

2. What would be the most likely cause for the hyponatremia noted in this patient on admission?

- Click on **Physician's Orders**.

3. What did the physician order on Tuesday at 1800 to treat this electrolyte imbalance?

4. Find Pablo Rodriguez's sodium and chloride levels for Wednesday at 0730. Was the physician's ordered treatment effective? Are there any changes in physician orders you might anticipate or suggest?

5. Hyponatremia can be associated with both hypovolemia (actual sodium loss) and hypervolemia (dilutional). Initially, in the Emergency Department, what do you think Pablo Rodriguez's volume status was? Explain.

- Click on **Return to Nurses' Station**.
- Click on **EPR**.
- Click on **Login**.
- Select **405** from the Patient drop-down menu and **Intake and Output** from the Category drop-down menu.

6. Below, record the intake and output shift totals for Tuesday at 2300 and Wednesday at 0700 for Pablo Rodriguez.

    Intake

    Output

7. Based on the above intake and output totals obtained after Pablo Rodriguez received IV replacement therapy, what factor(s) do you think may be contributing to the persistent hyponatremia? Explain your answer.

8. What other laboratory tests might be useful to more accurately determine the patient's hydration status? (*Hint:* See Chapter 11 in your textbook.)

- Click on **Return to Nurses' Station**.
- Click on **405** at the bottom of your screen.
- Click on **Patient Care** and then on **Physical Assessment**.
- Complete a physical assessment on Pablo Rodriguez by clicking on the body system categories (yellow buttons) and subcategories (green buttons).

9. Document findings from your physical assessment of Pablo Rodriguez that are indicative of hyponatremia.

Cardiovascular

Respiratory

Neuromuscular

Gastrointestinal

- Click on **Chart** and then **405**.
- Click on **Nursing Admission**.

10. What other factors could be causing or contributing to the manifestations documented in question 9?

11. Based on your answers to questions 9 and 10, what conclusion can you make regarding these clinical manifestations and Pablo Rodriguez's sodium levels?

12. What other clinical manifestations of hyponatremia might you expect to find in other patients with this electrolyte imbalance? (*Hint:* See Chapter 11 in your textbook.)

13. If Pablo Rodriguez's sodium level were 120 (severe hyponatremia), how would the treatment vary?

Exercise 3

Virtual Hospital Activity

60 minutes

- Sign in to work at Pacific View Regional Hospital for Period of Care 3. (*Note:* If you are already in the virtual hospital from a previous exercise, click on **Leave the Floor** and then on **Restart the Program** to get to the sign-in window.)
- From the Patient List, select Pablo Rodriguez (Room 405).
- Click on **Go to Nurses' Station**.
- Click on **Chart** and then on **405**.
- Click on **Laboratory Reports**.

1. What was Pablo Rodriguez's calcium level on admission to the Emergency Department on Tuesday evening?

2. How would you best describe this calcium level?

3. What was his phosphorus level during the same time frame?

4. How does this relate to his calcium level? Explain the pathophysiologic rationale supporting your answer.

- Click on **History and Physical**.

5. What would be the most likely cause for Pablo Rodriguez's calcium level?

6. Match each type of serum calcium imbalance with its potential cause. (*Note:* Each imbalance may be used more than once.)

Potential Cause

_____ Vitamin D deficiency

_____ Hyperthyroidism

_____ Hyperparathyroidism

_____ Excessive intake of phosphorous containing foods

_____ Kidney disease

Serum Calcium Imbalance

a. Hypercalcemia

b. Hypocalcemia

- Click on **Physician's Orders**.

7. What medication did the Emergency Department physician order in response to Pablo Rodriguez's serum calcium levels?

- Click on **Return to Nurses' Station**.
- Click on the **Drug Guide** on the counter.

8. Describe the mechanism of action of the medication you identified in question 7.

9. What nursing assessments are appropriate related to the administration of this medication?

- Click on **Return to Nurses' Station**.
- Click on **Chart** and then on **405**.
- Click on **Laboratory Reports**.

10. What were Pablo Rodriguez's calcium and phosphorus levels this morning (Wednesday at 0730)?

11. Was the prescribed medication effective? Is the patient out of danger?

- Click on **Return to Nurses' Station**.
- Click on **Kardex** and then on **405**.

12. What IV fluids is Pablo Rodriguez receiving?

13. What is the purpose of IV hydration in relation to serum calcium levels?

14. Is this the normal solution you would expect to administer to a patient with hypercalcemia? If not, what solution would you expect and why?

- Click on **Return to Nurses' Station**.
- Click on **MAR** and then on **405**.

15. What medication is scheduled to be administered at 1500?

16. What electrolyte imbalance will this medication correct? Explain your answer.

17. What nursing assessments must be completed before this drug is administered?

18. Do you have any concerns about administering this drug at this specific time? (*Hint:* Check the patient's gastrointestinal [GI] history on admission.)

- Click on **Return to Nurses' Station**.
- Go to Pablo Rodriguez's room by clicking on **405**.
- Click on **Patient Care** and then on **Physical Assessment**.
- Complete a physical assessment on Pablo Rodriguez by clicking on the body system categories (yellow buttons) and subcategories (green buttons).
- Click on **Take Vital Signs**.

19. Document the findings of your assessment, focusing on the areas listed below.

Cardiovascular

Respiratory

Neuromuscular

Gastrointestinal

20. Is Pablo Rodriguez demonstrating any clinical manifestations of hypercalcemia? If yes, describe the pathophysiologic basis for the symptoms. If not, explain why not.

21. If Pablo Rodriguez's calcium level were 12.5, what other clinical manifestations might the nurse expect to find? Select all that apply.

_____   Cardiac dysrhythmias

_____   Tachycardia

_____   Bradycardia

_____   Cyanosis

_____   Flushed skin

_____   Pallor

_____   Confusion

_____   Profound muscle weakness

_____   Hyperreflexia

_____   Decreased GI motility

_____   Diarrhea

22. Based on your vascular assessment of Pablo Rodriguez, what complication of hypercalcemia must the nurse vigilantly assess for? Explain.

23. After successful treatment of Pablo Rodriguez, the nurse must be alert for overcorrection of the electrolyte imbalance. For what clinical manifestations should the nurse monitor this patient related to hypocalcemia and hyperphosphatemia?

Acid-Base Imbalance

Reading Assignment: Assessment and Care of Patients with Problems of Acid-Base Balance
(Chapter 12)

Patients: Jacquline Catanazaro, Room 402
Patricia Newman, Room 406

Goal: To utilize the nursing process to competently care for patients with acid-base imbalances.

Objectives:

1. Describe the pathophysiologic basis of the acid-base imbalance noted in two patients.
2. Identify specific etiologic factor(s) related to respiratory acidosis in two patients.
3. Assess two patients for clinical manifestations related to respiratory acidosis.
4. Describe appropriate nursing interventions to use when caring for specific patients with respiratory acidosis.
5. Evaluate the effectiveness of medication prescribed to treat acid-base imbalances.

In this lesson you will assess, plan, and implement care for two patients with an acid-base imbalance. Jacquline Catanazaro is a 45-year-old female admitted with exacerbation of asthma and schizophrenia. Patricia Newman is a 61-year-old female admitted with pneumonia and a 12-year history of emphysema. You will begin this lesson by first reviewing the general concepts of acid-base balance as presented in your textbook.

Exercise 1

Writing Activity

10 minutes

1. Match each term with its corresponding definition. (*Hint:* See Chapter 12 in your textbook.)

Term	Definition
_____ Acid	a. A measure of the body fluid's free hydrogen ion level
_____ Base	b. Substance that binds free hydrogen ions in solution
_____ pH	c. Substance that releases hydrogen ions when dissolved in water

2. Identify and describe three methods of acid-base homeostasis. Indicate the type of defense and the associated mechanisms of action.

First line of defense

Second line of defense

Third line of defense

Exercise 2

Virtual Hospital Activity

45 minutes

- Sign in to work at Pacific View Regional Hospital for Period of Care 1. (*Note:* If you are already in the virtual hospital from a previous exercise, click on **Leave the Floor** and then on **Restart the Program** to get to the sign-in window.)
- From the Patient List, select Jacquline Catanazaro (Room 402).
- Click on **Go to Nurses' Station**.
- Click on **Chart** and then on **402**.
- Click on **History and Physical**.

   1. Is there anything in Jacquline Catanazaro's history that would put her at risk for an acid-base imbalance?

- Click on **Return to Nurses' Station**.
- Click on **402** at the bottom of your screen.
- Click on **Patient Care** and then on **Nurse-Client Interactions**.
- Select and view the video titled **0730: Intervention—Airway**. (*Note:* Check the virtual clock to see whether enough time has elapsed. You can use the fast-forward feature to advance the time by 2-minute intervals if the video is not yet available. Then click again on **Patient Care** and on **Nurse-Client Interactions** to refresh the screen.)

   2. Based on Jacquline Catanazaro's history, what would the nurse expect to be causing her respiratory distress?

   3. Why is the nurse waiting until after the arterial blood gases (ABGs) are drawn to give the patient a nebulizer treatment?

- Click on **Chart** and then on **402**.
- Click on **Laboratory Reports**.

4. Document the results of Jacquline Catanazaro's ABG on Monday at 1030.

   pH

   PaO_2

   $PaCO_2$

   O_2 sat

   Bicarb

5. Document the results of Jacquline Catanazaro's ABG on Wednesday at 0730.

   pH

   PaO_2

   $PaCO_2$

   O_2 sat

   Bicarb

6. How would you interpret the results documented in questions 4 and 5? Is the acid-base imbalance compensated or uncompensated (fully or partially)? Explain your answer.

7. Based on the acute aspect of Jacquline Catanazaro's respiratory difficulties, what lines of defense would you expect to be working to compensate for her respiratory acidosis?

8. If the patient's electrolyte results were available, what might you expect her potassium levels to be? Provide a rationale for your answer. (*Hint:* See Chapter 12 in your textbook.)

9. Based on Jacquline Catanazaro's medical diagnosis, what is the underlying pathophysiologic problem leading to the respiratory acidosis? (*Hint:* See Chapter 12 in your textbook.)

- Click on **Return to Room 402**.
- Click on **Patient Care** and then on **Physical Assessment**.
- Complete a physical assessment for Jacquline Catanazaro by clicking on the body system categories (yellow buttons) and subcategories (green buttons).

10. Record the findings of your physical assessment below.

Mental status

Musculoskeletal

Cardiovascular

Respiratory

Integumentary

11. Are there any clinical manifestations of respiratory acidosis? If so, please describe. If not, how do you explain?

- Click on **Take Vital Signs**.

12. What is the patient's respiratory rate? How does this correlate with her respiratory acidosis?

13. If Jacquline Catanazaro's pH were 7.2, how might her physical assessment differ? Document the expected clinical manifestations of respiratory acidosis below.

Neurologic

Musculoskeletal

Cardiovascular

Respiratory

Integumentary

- Click on **Chart**.
- Click on **402** for Jacquline Catanazaro's chart.
- Click on **Physician's Orders**.

14. Look at the most recent physician's orders. What medication is ordered to treat the respiratory acidosis? What is the medication's underlying mechanism of action to correct the acidosis? (*Hint:* See Drug Guide.)

- Click on **Return to Room 402**.
- Click on **Leave the Floor**.
- Click on **Restart the Program**.
- Sign in to work at Pacific View Regional Hospital for Period of Care 2.
- From the Patient List, select Jacquline Catanazaro (Room 402).
- Click on **Go to Nurses' Station**.
- Click on **Chart** and then on **402**.
- Click on **Laboratory Reports**. Scroll down to review the results for Wed 1000.

15. Look at the ABGs drawn at 1000. Interpret the ABGs. Was the treatment effective?

Exercise 3

Virtual Hospital Activity

45 minutes

- Sign in to work at Pacific View Regional Hospital for Period of Care 1. (*Note:* If you are already in the virtual hospital from a previous exercise, click on **Leave the Floor** and then on **Restart the Program** to get to the sign-in window.)
- From the Patient List, select Patricia Newman (Room 406).
- Click on **Go to Nurses' Station**.
- Click on **Chart** and then on **406**.
- Click on **History and Physical**.

1. Is there anything in Patricia Newman's history that would put her at risk for an acid-base imbalance?

- Click on **Laboratory Reports**.

2. Document the results of Patricia Newman's two most recent ABGs (Tuesday 2300 and Wednesday 0500) below. Include pH, PaO_2, $PaCO_2$, O_2 sat, and bicarb.

   Tuesday 2300

   Wednesday 0500

3. How would you interpret the results you recorded in the previous table? Is the acid-base imbalance compensated or uncompensated (fully or partially)? Explain your answer.

4. Based on the chronic aspect of Patricia Newman's respiratory difficulties, what lines of defense would you expect to be working to compensate for the respiratory acidosis?

5. Based on the ABG results, has Patricia Newman's condition improved or worsened since admission the evening before?

• Click on **Nurse's Notes**.

6. Read the notes for Wednesday 0730. Describe the actions taken by the nurse. Are they appropriate or not? Explain you answer.

7. What additional actions do you think would be appropriate at this time?

• Click on **Laboratory Reports**.

8. The patient's serum potassium level is _____ mEq/L.

9. How would you explain the patient's hypokalemia in relation to respiratory acidosis? (*Hint:* See the **Drug Guide** and Chapter 12 in your textbook.)

10. Based on Patricia Newman's medical diagnosis, what is the underlying pathophysiologic problem leading to the respiratory acidosis? How does that differ from Jacquline Catanazaro's problem in the previous exercise of this lesson? (*Hint:* See Chapter 12 in your textbook.)

- Click on **Return to Nurses' Station**.
- Click on **406** at the bottom of your screen.
- Click on **Patient Care** and then on **Physical Assessment**.
- Complete a physical assessment for Patricia Newman by clicking on the body categories (yellow buttons) and subcategories (green buttons).
- Click on **Take Vital Signs**.

11. Document the findings of your physical assessment below.

Mental status

Musculoskeletal

Cardiovascular

Respiratory

Integumentary

12. Does Patricia Newman demonstrate any clinical manifestations of respiratory acidosis? If so, please describe. If not, explain why not.

13. What nursing interventions could you, as a graduate nurse, plan and implement to improve Patricia Newman's acid-base balance and prevent complications?

LESSON 7

Perioperative Care

Reading Assignment: Care of Preoperative Patients (Chapter 14)
Care of Postoperative Patients (Chapter 16)
Care of Patients with Hematologic Problems (Chapter 40)

Patients: Piya Jordan, Room 403
Clarence Hughes, Room 404

Goal: To utilize the nursing process to competently care for perioperative patients.

Objectives:

1. Document a complete history and physical on a preoperative patient.
2. Identify appropriate rationales for preoperative orders on an assigned patient.
3. Evaluate completeness of preoperative teaching on a patient scheduled for surgery.
4. Document a focused assessment on a patient transferred from the postanesthesia care unit (PACU) to a medical-surgical unit.
5. Plan appropriate interventions to prevent postoperative complications in an assigned patient.
6. Utilize the nursing process to correctly administer scheduled and prn medications to an assigned patient.

In this lesson you will learn the essentials of caring for patients in both the preoperative and postoperative stages of surgery. You will document assessments and plan, implement, and evaluate care given. Piya Jordan is a 68-year-old female admitted with nausea and vomiting for 3 days. Clarence Hughes is a 73-year-old male admitted for an elective knee replacement.

Exercise 1

Virtual Hospital Activity

45 minutes

- Sign in to work at Pacific View Regional Hospital for Period of Care 1. (*Note:* If you are already in the virtual hospital from a previous exercise, click on **Leave the Floor** and then on **Restart the Program** to get to the sign-in window.)
- From the Patient List, select Piya Jordan (Room 403).
- Click on **Go to Nurses' Station**.
- Click on **Chart** and then on **403**.
- Click on **Emergency Department** and review the record.

1. What complaints (problems) brought Piya Jordan to the Emergency Department?

2. What were her primary and secondary admitting diagnoses on admission?

- Click on **Nursing Admission**.
- Click on **History and Physical**.

3. Which findings from the preoperative health history increase Piya Jordan's risk for surgical complications? Select all that apply. (*Hint:* See Table 14-3.)

_____ Age 68 years

_____ Arthritis in knees

_____ Atrial fibrillation

_____ Celecoxib 300 mg every 12 hours

_____ Digoxin 0.125 mg daily

_____ Stress incontinence

_____ Warfarin 5 mg daily

- Now click on **Laboratory Report**.

4. Record Piya Jordan's CBC results from Monday at 2200. Insert an asterisk after any results that are abnormal.

   White blood cell count (WBC)

   Red blood cell count (RBC)

   Hemoglobin

   Hematocrit

   Platelets

5. Record Piya Jordan's electrolyte results from Monday at 2200. Insert an asterisk after any results that are abnormal.

   Glucose

   Sodium

   Potassium

6. Record Piya Jordan's renal results from Monday at 2200. Insert an asterisk after any results that are abnormal.

   Blood urea nitrogen (BUN)

   Creatinine

7. Record Piya Jordan's urinalysis results from Monday at 2200. Insert an asterisk after any results that are abnormal.

   Urine glucose

   Blood

   Protein

   Leukocytes

8. Record Piya Jordan's coagulation test results from Monday at 2200. Insert an asterisk after any results that are abnormal.

   Prothrombin time (PT)

   International normalized ratio (INR)

9. Record Piya Jordan's blood type results from Tuesday at 0630.

10. Are any of Piya Jordan's laboratory results abnormal or of concern for a patient preparing to undergo surgery? Explain. (*Hint:* See Chapter 14 in your textbook.)

- Click on **Surgical Reports**.

11. Which best describes the type of surgery Piya Jordan had performed?
    a. Diagnostic
    b. Curative
    c. Restorative
    d. Palliative
    e. Cosmetic

12. Piya Jordan is 68 years of age. Her age increases her risk for the development of postoperative complications. For each body system below, list the age-related physiologic changes that increase her risks for complications and may delay her recovery. Then identify one to two nursing interventions that may be implemented to reduce complications.

Cardiovascular system

Respiratory system

Renal system

Neurologic system

Integumentary system

13. When reviewing the medication list of a patient scheduled for surgery, which medication types are associated with an increased risk for complications? Select all that apply.

_____ Antibiotics

_____ Nonsteroidal antiinflammatory agents

_____ Anticoagulants

_____ Diuretics

_____ Antihypertensives

_____ Tricyclic antidepressants

Exercise 2

Virtual Hospital Activity

30 minutes

- Sign in to work at Pacific View Regional Hospital for Period of Care 1. (*Note:* If you are already in the virtual hospital from a previous exercise, click on **Leave the Floor** and then on **Restart the Program** to get to the sign-in window.)
- From the Patient List, select Piya Jordan (Room 403).
- Click on **Go to Nurses' Station**.
- Click on **Chart** and then on **403**.
- Click on **Consents**.

1. For what procedure(s) has Piya Jordan given written consent?

2. Who is responsible for providing detailed information about the procedure(s) for which Piya Jordan has given consent?

3. Which are nursing responsibilities in regard to obtaining informed consent? Select all that apply. (*Hint:* See Chapter 14 in your textbook.)

   _____ Clarify information presented by the physician

   _____ Witness patient signature

   _____ Provide detailed information about the risks and benefits of the planned procedure

   _____ Ensure the patient has complete understanding about the procedure

- Now click on **Physician's Orders**.

4. Look at the orders for Tuesday 0130. What consent was ordered?

LESSON 7—PERIOPERATIVE CARE   109

5. By when does this consent need to be obtained?

6. What is the purpose of the mineral oil enema that was ordered to be given to Piya Jordan?

7. What diet has the physician ordered preoperatively? What is the purpose for this diet order?

8. The American Society of Anesthesiologists recommends an NPO time of at least _____ hours

   for easily digested solid foods and _____ hours for clear liquids before surgery.

9. What is the rationale for giving Piya Jordan a unit of fresh frozen plasma preoperatively?
   (*Hint:* See Chapter 40 in your textbook.)

10. How long before surgery can an autologous blood transfusion be obtained? What is an advantage of
    this type of blood transfusion?

11. What is the rationale for ordering a dose of cefotetan on call (to be hung and administered upon
    transport to the OR) to the operating room for Piya Jordan? Is this a safe order to administer to her?
    Explain why or why not. (*Hint:* See Chapter 14 in your textbook.)

- Click on **Surgical Reports**. Scroll down to the Preoperative Checklist.

12. Using Table 14-4 in your textbook, list the items that should be considered when planning preoperative teaching. Place an asterisk by those items that were *NOT* covered, according to Piya Jordan's Preoperative Checklist.

Exercise 3

Virtual Hospital Activity

45 minutes

Clarence Hughes' scheduled surgery has been completed. You will be reviewing the care already given to him and planning and evaluating care for him during the immediate postoperative period.

- Sign in to work at Pacific View Regional Hospital for Period of Care 1. (*Note:* If you are already in the virtual hospital from a previous exercise, click on **Leave the Floor** and then on **Restart the Program** to get to the sign-in window.)
- From the Patient List, select Clarence Hughes (Room 404).
- Click on **Go to Nurses' Station**.
- Click on **EPR** and then on **Login**.
- Select **404** from the Patient drop-down menu.
- From the Category drop-down menu, select and review **Vital Signs**, **Respiratory**, **Neurologic**, **Integumentary**, **IV**, **Wounds and Drains**, and any other EPR categories necessary to answer the following question.

1. A postoperative patient requires an immediate focused assessment on arrival to the medical-surgical nursing unit. Document the assessment findings recorded by the nurse on Sunday at 1600 when Clarence Hughes arrived on the medical-surgical unit. Be sure to check the following key assessment areas in the EPR: Respiratory, Neurologic, Vital Signs, IV, and Wounds and Drains. (*Note:* If information is not explicitly available in the EPR, list where information can be found based on codes.)

Respiratory

Neurologic

Vital Signs

IV

Wounds and Drains

2. How frequently did the nurse assess Clarence Hughes' vital signs after his arrival on the unit? How often do you think they should be assessed? (*Hint:* See Chapter 16 in your textbook.)

- Still in the EPR, select **Intake and Output** from the Category drop-down menu.

3. Record Clarence Hughes' intake and output for the past 3 days by documenting the intake (I) and output (O) totals for each of the times below.

Sunday 2300	I: _____	O: _____
Monday 0700	I: _____	O: _____
Monday 1500	I: _____	O: _____
Monday 2300	I: _____	O: _____
Tuesday 0700	I: _____	O: _____
Tuesday 1500	I: _____	O: _____
Tuesday 2300	I: _____	O: _____
Wednesday 0700	I: _____	O: _____

4. Which is greater—Clarence Hughes' intake or output? By how much? Is this expected?

5. What are the possible consequences if this trend in fluid balance continues?

- Click on **Exit EPR**.
- Click on **Chart** and then on **404**.
- Click on **Physician's Orders**.

6. Look at the physician's postoperative orders written on Sunday at 1600. What is ordered to prevent postoperative atelectasis and/or pneumonia?

7. The physician prescribed enoxaparin. What is the purpose of this medication?
   a. Prevention of infection
   b. Prevention of deep vein thrombosis
   c. Pain management
   d. Reduction of postoperative constipation

8. When preparing to administer enoxaparin, the review of which laboratory test result is most important?
   a. Calcium level
   b. Complete blood cell count
   c. Urinalysis
   d. Liver enzymes

9. When reviewing Clarence Hughes' health history, which finding, if noted, would be cause for concern with the administration of enoxaparin?
   a. Renal impairment
   b. Immunodeficiency
   c. History of latex allergy
   d. Anemia

10. What wound care is ordered on Sunday?

11. Explain how and when to perform the ordered wound care.

- Click on **Return to Nurses' Station** and then on **404**.
- Inside Clarence Hughes' room, click on **Take Vital Signs**. Review these results.
- Click on **Clinical Alerts**.
- Click on **Patient Care** and then on **Nurse-Client Interactions**.
- Select and view the video titled **0735: Empathy**. (*Note:* Check the virtual clock to see whether enough time has elapsed. You can use the fast-forward feature to advance the time by 2-minute intervals if the video is not yet available. Then click again on **Patient Care** and on **Nurse-Client Interactions** to refresh the screen.)

12. What is Clarence Hughes' major concern at this point?

- Now click on **Medication Room**.
- From the Medication Room, click on **MAR** to determine the medications that Clarence Hughes is ordered to receive at 0800 and any appropriate prn medications you may want to administer. (*Note:* You may click on **Review MAR** at any time to verify correct medication order. Click on the correct room number within the MAR. Remember to look at the patient name on the MAR to make sure you have the correct patient's record. Click on **Return to Medication Room** after reviewing the correct MAR.)
- Click on **Unit Dosage**.
- Click on drawer **404**.
- From the list of available medications in the top window, select the medication(s) you would like to administer. After each medication you select, click on **Put Medication on Tray**.
- When you have finished putting your selected medications on the tray, click on **Close Drawer**.
- Click on **View Medication Room**.
- This time, click on **Automated System**. Your name and password will automatically appear. Click on **Login**.
- In box 1, select the correct patient; in box 2, choose the appropriate Automated System Drawer for this patient. Then click on **Open Drawer**.
- From the list of available medications, select the medication(s) you would like to administer. For each one selected, click on **Put Medication on Tray**. When you are finished, click on **Close Drawer**.
- Click on **View Medication Room**.
- From the Medication Room, click on **Preparation** and then highlight the medication you want to administer. Click on **Prepare**.
- Wait for the Preparation Wizard to appear; then provide any information requested.
- Click on **Next**, choose the correct patient to administer this medication to, and click on **Finish**.
- Repeat the previous three steps until you have prepared all the medications you want to administer.
- You can click on **Review Your Medications** and then on **Return to Medication Room** when you are ready. Once you are back in the Medication Room, you may go directly to Clarence Hughes' room by clicking on **404** at bottom of the screen.
- Administer the medication, utilizing the six rights of medication administration. After you have collected the appropriate assessment data and are ready for administration, click on **Patient Care** and then on **Medication Administration**. Verify that the correct patient and medication(s) appear in the left-hand window. Then click the down arrow next to Select.

- From the drop-down menu, select **Administer** and complete the Administration Wizard by providing any information requested. When the Wizard stops asking for information, click on **Administer to Patient**. Specify **Yes** when asked whether this administration should be recorded in the MAR. Finally, click on **Finish**.

Now let's see how you did!

- Click on **Leave the Floor** at the bottom of your screen. From the Floor Menu, click on **Look at Your Preceptor's Evaluation** and then click on **Medication Scorecard**.

13. Note below whether or not you correctly administered the appropriate medication(s). If not, why do you think you were incorrect? According to Table C in this scorecard, what resources should be used and what important assessments should be completed before administering the medication(s)? Did you utilize these resources and perform these assessments correctly?

Osteoarthritis and Total Knee Replacement

Reading Assignment: Care of Preoperative Patients (Chapter 14)
Care of Patients with Arthritis and Other Connective Tissue Diseases
(Chapter 18)

Patient: Clarence Hughes, Room 404

Goal: To utilize the nursing process to competently care for patients with arthritis.

Objectives:

1. Describe the clinical manifestations of osteoarthritis (OA).
2. Plan and implement treatment for a patient with OA.
3. Document a focused assessment on a postoperative patient who has undergone a total knee arthroplasty/total knee replacement (TKA/TKR).
4. Plan appropriate interventions to prevent complications related to a TKA/TKR.
5. Identify and provide rationales for collaborative care measures used to treat a patient after a TKA/TKR.

In this lesson you will learn the essentials of caring for a patient who has had a TKA/TKR as treatment for debilitating OA. You will document assessments and plan, implement, and evaluate care. Clarence Hughes is a 73-year-old male admitted for an elective knee replacement. You will begin this lesson by first reviewing the general concepts of OA as presented in your textbook.

Exercise 1

Writing Activity

15 minutes

1. Briefly describe the pathophysiology of OA. (*Hint:* See Chapter 18 in your textbook.)

2. Which are considered to be causative factors related to the occurrence of primary osteoarthritis? Select all that apply.

_____ Aging

_____ Genetic changes

_____ Obesity

_____ Joint trauma

_____ Autoimmune factors

_____ Medication usage

3. What are the clinical manifestations of OA?

4. What laboratory and/or radiographic testing is used in the diagnosis of OA? (*Hint:* See Chapter 18 in your textbook.)

5. How do primary and secondary osteoarthritis differ?

6. What metabolic disorders are associated with the development of osteoarthritis? Select all that apply.

_____   Diabetes mellitus

_____   Sickle cell anemia

_____   Hypertension

_____   Right-sided heart failure

_____   Paget's disease

_____   Hemophilia

Exercise 2

Virtual Hospital Activity

40 minutes

- Sign in to work at Pacific View Regional Hospital for Period of Care 1. (*Note:* If you are already in the virtual hospital from a previous exercise, click on **Leave the Floor** and then on **Restart the Program** to get to the sign-in window.)
- From the Patient List, select Clarence Hughes (Room 404).
- Click on **Go to Nurses' Station**.
- Click on **Chart** and then on **404**.
- Click on **History and Physical**.

1. According to the Plan at the bottom of the History and Physical, why was Clarence Hughes admitted to the hospital?

2. Describe the symptoms that brought Clarence Hughes to this point.

3. According to the History and Physical, what medications and/or treatments were used to treat Clarence Hughes before he elected to have surgery?

4. Which type of osteoarthritis does Clarence Hughes have?
   a. Primary
   b. Secondary

5. Explain the rationale for performing a TKA/TKR on this patient.

- Click on **Surgical Reports**.

6. How does the report of operation describe the surgical procedure performed on Clarence Hughes?

7. How would the minimally invasive surgical procedure differ?

8. What was Clarence Hughes' estimated blood loss (EBL)?

- Click on **Physician's Orders**.
- Scroll down to read the orders for Sunday 1600.

9. What frequent assessments are ordered? Describe specifically how these assessments are completed and what the nurse is looking for.

10. What type of surgical drain has been placed in Clarence Hughes' incision?

- Click on **Return to Nurses' Station**.
- Click on **EPR** and **Login**.
- Select **404** from the Patient drop-down menu and **Intake and Output** from the Category drop-down menu.

11. List the amount of drainage recorded for drain 1 (Hemovac) in the immediate postoperative period.

    Sunday 2300

    Monday 0700

12. _____ The amount of drainage to Hemovac has increased since Clarence Hughes was admitted to the unit. (True or False)

- Click on **Return to Nurses' Station**.
- Click on **Chart** and then on **404**.
- Click on **Physician's Notes**.
- Scroll down to read the note for Mon 0730.

13. What is the status of the Hemovac at this time? How does the physician describe the dressing and/or amount of drainage?

- Click on **Physician's Orders**.
- Scroll down to read the orders for Monday 0715.

14. What is ordered to be applied to the operative knee? Explain the basic use of this device. (*Hint:* See Chapter 18 in your textbook.)

15. According to the physician's notes, how should Clarence Hughes' operative leg be positioned when the device that you identified in question 14 is not in use? Are there any other positioning precautions that should be taken into consideration? (*Hint:* See Chapter 18 in your textbook.)

* Click on **Laboratory Reports**.

16. What was Clarence Hughes' hemoglobin (Hgb) and hematocrit (Hct) values on Monday at 0600 and Tuesday at 0600?

    Monday 0600

    Tuesday 0600

* Click on **Return to Nurse's Station**.
* Click on **EPR**. Click on **Login**.
* Select **404** from the Patient drop-down menu and **Intake and Output** from the Category drop-down menu.

17. Calculate the intravenous (IV) fluid intake from the time that Clarence Hughes was admitted to the floor until Tuesday at 0600 using the total intake for Sunday 2300, Monday 0700, and Monday 2300. Then determine the total blood loss from surgery (EBL) plus the drainage you recorded for question 11.

    Total fluid intake

    Total blood loss

18. Based on the information gathered in question 17, what might be the explanation for the drop in Hgb and Hct?

* Click on **Return to Nurse's Station**.
* Click on **Chart** and then on **404**.
* Click on **Physician's Orders**. Scroll to and review the order for Tue 1000.

19. What was ordered to correct the decreased hemoglobin?

Exercise 3

Virtual Hospital Activity

45 minutes

- Sign in to work at Pacific View Regional Hospital for Period of Care 1. (*Note:* If you are already in the virtual hospital from a previous exercise, click on **Leave the Floor** and then on **Restart the Program** to get to the sign-in window.)
- From the Patient List, select Clarence Hughes (Room 404).
- Click on **Get Report**.

1. What are your concerns for Clarence Hughes after receiving this report?

- Click on **Go to Nurses' Station**.
- Click on **404** at the bottom of your screen.
- Click on **Patient Care** and then on **Physical Assessment**.
- Complete a focused assessment by clicking on the body system categories (yellow buttons) and subcategories (green buttons).

2. Document the findings of your focused assessment for the integumentary, musculoskeletal, gastrointestinal, and respiratory systems below and on the next page.

Integumentary

Musculoskeletal

Neurovascular

Gastrointestinal

Respiratory

- Click on **Clinical Alerts**.

3. Based on the findings of your physical assessment and the information in the clinical alert, what would be your priority interventions?

- Click on **Medication Room**.
- Click on **MAR** to determine prn medications that have been ordered for Clarence Hughes to address his constipation and pain. (*Note:* You may click on **Review MAR** at any time to verify correct medication order. Click on the correct room number within the MAR. Remember to look at the patient name on the MAR to make sure you have the correct patient's record. Click on **Return to Medication Room** after reviewing the correct MAR.)
- Click on **Unit Dosage** and then click on drawer **404**.
- Select the medications you would like to administer. After each selection, click on **Put Medication on Tray**. When you are finished selecting medications, click on **Close Drawer**.
- Click on **View Medication Room**.
- Click on **Automated System** and then click on **Login**.
- On the next screen, specify the correct patient and drawer location.
- Select the medication you would like to administer and click on **Put Medication on Tray**. Repeat this process if you wish to administer other medications from the Automated System.
- When you are finished, click on **Close Drawer**. At the bottom right corner of the next screen, click on **View Medication Room**.
- From the Medication Room, click on **Preparation** (or on the preparation tray).
- From the list of medications on your tray, choose the correct medication to administer. Click on **Prepare**.

- Supply the information that the Preparation Wizard requests.
- Click on **Next**, specify the correct patient to administer this medication to, and then click on **Finish**.
- Repeat the previous three steps until all medications that you want to administer are prepared.
- You can click on **Review Your Medications** and then on **Return to Medication Room** when ready. Once you are back in the Medication Room, you may go directly to Clarence Hughes' room by clicking on **404** at the bottom of the screen.
- Administer the medication, utilizing the six rights of medication administration. After you have collected the appropriate assessment data and are ready for administration, click on **Patient Care** and then on **Medication Administration**. Verify that the correct patient and medication(s) appear in the left-hand window. Click the down arrow next to Select. From the drop-down menu, select **Administer** and complete the Administration Wizard by providing any information requested. When the Wizard stops asking for information, click on **Administer to Patient**. Specify **Yes** when asked whether this administration should be recorded in the MAR. Finally, click on **Finish**. You will evaluate your performance in this area at the end of this exercise (see question 14).

4. What is missing on Clarence Hughes' order for oxycodone with acetaminophen? What measures need to be taken?

5. Based on the knowledge that most antacids frequently decrease absorption of other medications when concurrently administered, what options might the nurse employ to ensure adequate absorption of pain medication? (*Hint:* Look in the Drug Guide.)

- Click on **Patient Care** and then on **Nurse-Client Interactions**.
- Select and view the video titled **0735: Empathy**. (*Note:* Check the virtual clock to see whether enough time has elapsed. You can use the fast-forward feature to advance the time by 2-minute intervals if the video is not yet available. Then click again on **Patient Care** and on **Nurse-Client Interactions** to refresh the screen.)

6. The nurse attempts to appear empathetic by offering to listen to the patient's concerns. Are her actions congruent with her verbal communication? Why or why not?

7. As a student nurse, what would you do differently?

8. Identify potential complications related to Clarence Hughes' postoperative status and measures that can be implemented to prevent them. Document your plan of care below.

- Click on **Chart** and then on **404**.
- Click on **Consultations**.

9. What is physical therapy (PT) doing for Clarence Hughes?

- Click on **Physician's Orders**.

10. What is the patient's activity order for Wednesday morning?

- Click on **Physician's Orders**. Scroll and review the order for Mon 0715.

11. What is Clarence Hughes' goal for CPM therapy today (postoperative day 3)?

- Click on **Nurse's Notes**. Review the notes for Wednesday and Tuesday.
- Click on **Nursing Admission**. Scroll to page 12 and review Clarence Hughes' home environment.

12. Based on the orders and the patient's activity and home environment, do you think the ambulation activity and the CPM goal are sufficient for this patient to be discharged tomorrow? Why or why not? (*Hint:* See Chapter 18 in your textbook.)

• Click on **Patient Education**.

13. What teaching should be completed for Clarence Hughes before his discharge?

14. In the absence of complications, total recovery after a TKA can be anticipated within what time period?
    a. 2 weeks
    b. 4 weeks
    c. 6 weeks
    d. 8 weeks

Now let's see how you did during your earlier medication administration!

• Click on **Leave the Floor**. From the Floor Menu, click on **Look at Your Preceptor's Evaluation** and then click on **Medication Scorecard**.

15. Disregard the report for the routine scheduled medications, and instead note below whether or not you correctly administered the appropriate prn medications. If not, why do you think you were incorrect? According to Table C in this scorecard, what resources should be used and what important assessments should be completed before administering these medications? Did you utilize these resources and perform these assessments correctly?

Cancer

Reading Assignment: Principles of Cancer Development (Chapter 21)
Care of Patients with Cancer (Chapter 22)
Care of Patients with Noninfectious Lower Respiratory Problems
(Chapter 30)

Patient: Pablo Rodriguez, Room 405

Goal: To utilize the nursing process to competently care for patients with cancer.

Objectives:

1. Describe the clinical manifestations of cancer.
2. Plan, implement, and evaluate treatment for a patient with cancer.
3. Recognize special needs of patients undergoing treatment for cancer.
4. Appropriately treat a patient's symptoms related to disease process and/or side effects of treatment.
5. Discuss medications prescribed for an assigned patient, including expected therapeutic effects as well as side effects and adverse effects.
6. Plan appropriate general interventions to prevent and/or treat complications related to chemotherapy.

In this lesson you will learn the essentials of caring for a patient diagnosed with cancer. You will collect data and assess, plan, implement, and evaluate care given. Pablo Rodriguez is a 71-year-old male admitted with advanced non-small cell lung carcinoma (NSCLC). You will begin this lesson by first reviewing the general concepts of cancer as presented in your textbook.

Exercise 1

Writing Activity

15 minutes

1. Match each term below with its corresponding definition.

Term	Definition
_____ Carcinogenesis	a. A substance that promotes or enhances growth of the initiated cancer cell
_____ Initiation	
	b. An irreversible event that can lead to cancer development
_____ Carcinogen	
	c. Another name for cancer development
_____ Promoter	
	d. Substance that changes the activity of a cell's gene so that the cell becomes a cancer cell
_____ Nadir	
	e. The time when bone marrow activity and white blood cell counts (WBCs) are at their lowest levels after chemotherapy

2. Match each type of therapy with the most accurate description.

Type of Therapy	Description
_____ Surgery	a. Uses high-energy radiation from gamma rays, radionuclides, or ionizing radiation beams to kill cancer cells, provide disease control, or relieve symptoms
_____ Radiation therapy	
	b. Often plays a part in the diagnosis and management of cancer. Used for prophylaxis, diagnosis, cure, control, palliation, assessment of treatment effectiveness, or tissue reconstruction
_____ Chemotherapy	
	c. Uses antineoplastic drugs to kill cancer cells and disrupt their cellular regulation

3. What are the common sites of metastasis for lung cancer? Select all that apply. (*Hint:* See Table 21-2 in your textbook.)

_____ Central nervous system

_____ Lymph nodes

_____ Bone

_____ Pancreas

_____ Brain

_____ Gastrointestinal (GI) tract

_____ Liver

4. List the warning signals associated with lung cancer. (*Hint:* See Table 30-5 in your textbook.)

Exercise 2

Virtual Hospital Activity

35 minutes

- Sign in to work at Pacific View Regional Hospital for Period of Care 1. (*Note:* If you are already in the virtual hospital from a previous exercise, click on **Leave the Floor** and then on **Restart the Program** to get to the sign-in window.)
- From the Patient List, select Pablo Rodriguez (Room 405).
- Click on **Go to Nurses' Station**.
- Click on **Chart** and then on **405** for Pablo Rodriguez's chart.
- Click on **History and Physical**.

1. What is Pablo Rodriguez's main diagnosis?

2. How long ago was he diagnosed?

3. What risk factor for lung cancer is documented on the History and Physical?

4. What other risk factors for lung cancer are described in your textbook? (*Hint:* See Chapter 30 in your textbook.)

5. What clinical manifestations documented in the physician's review of systems are related to the disease process of lung cancer?

6. What treatment has Pablo Rodriguez received so far?

7. How long ago did he receive his last chemotherapy?

- Click on **Emergency Department**. Scroll down to review the Emergency Department physician's progress notes for Tue at 1800.

8. The Emergency Department physician notes that Pablo Rodriguez had a chest x-ray and bronchoscopy 1 year ago. Which type of cancer were the findings of the bronchoscopy consistent with? Is this the same type of cancer as was noted by the admitting physician in the History and Physical?

Exercise 3

Virtual Hospital Activity

30 minutes

- Sign in to work at Pacific View Regional Hospital for Period of Care 1. (*Note:* If you are already in the virtual hospital from a previous exercise, click on **Leave the Floor** and then on **Restart the Program** to get to the sign-in window.)
- From the Patient List, select Pablo Rodriguez (Room 405).
- Click on **Get Report**.

1. Which of the problems noted in the shift report were unresolved as of the beginning of Period of Care 1?

- Click on **Go to Nurses' Station**.
- Click on **Chart** and then on **405**.
- Click on **Nurse's Notes**.

2. Look at the note for Wednesday at 0415. How did the nurse respond to Pablo Rodriguez's complaints? Were the nurse's actions appropriate?

3. How might you have responded differently?

- Click on **Return to Nurses' Station**.
- Click on **405** at the bottom of your screen.
- Click on **Patient Care** and then on **Nurse-Client Interactions**.
- Select and view the video titled **0730: Symptom Management**. (*Note:* Check the virtual clock to see whether enough time has elapsed. You can use the fast-forward feature to advance the time by 2-minute intervals if the video is not yet available. Then click again on **Patient Care** and on **Nurse-Client Interactions** to refresh the screen.)

4. What are Pablo Rodriguez's two primary concerns at this point?

5. What assessment should you perform before treating the patient's complaint of nausea?

- Click on **MAR**; then select tab **405** to access Pablo Rodriguez's record.

6. What medications are ordered to manage the patient's nausea?

7. What might the nurse question regarding these medication orders?

- Click on **Return to Room 405**.
- Click on **Chart** and then on **405**.
- Click on **Nursing Admission**.

8. What is the patient's weight in pounds? What is this in kilograms?

- Click on **Return to Room 405**.
- Click on the **Drug** icon in the lower left corner of the screen.

9. Using the information from the Drug Guide and the patient's weight, determine the maximum dose that Pablo Rodriguez can receive of metoclopramide within a 24-hour period for prevention of chemotherapy-induced nausea and vomiting and for postoperative nausea and vomiting. List only the maximum doses for the indications specified below.

Prevention of cancer chemotherapy–
induced nausea and vomiting

Postoperative nausea and vomiting

10. Calculate the maximum amount of metoclopramide Pablo Rodriguez could receive per 24 hours as ordered. Is this within the dosage guidelines? Is there any reason to be concerned about Pablo Rodriguez receiving this dosage over long periods of time?

11. What are the possible ramifications of giving high doses of this drug?

12. What are the ramifications of *not* administering this drug for Pablo Rodriguez's complaint of nausea?

13. If the nurse administers the prn dose for this drug at 0730, what should be done with the regularly scheduled 0800 dose?

Exercise 4

Virtual Hospital Activity

40 minutes

- Sign in to work at Pacific View Regional Hospital for Period of Care 2. (*Note:* If you are already in the virtual hospital from a previous exercise, click on **Leave the Floor** and then on **Restart the Program** to get to the sign-in window.)
- From the Patient List, select Pablo Rodriguez (Room 405).
- Click on **Go to Nurses' Station**.
- Click on **Chart** and then on **405**.
- Click on **Emergency Department**.

1. What is Pablo Rodriguez's chief complaint on admission to the Emergency Department? How is this related to his cancer? (*Hint:* See Chapter 22 in your textbook. Review the Emergency Department physician's note for Tue at 1800.)

- Click on **Return to Nurses' Station**.
- Click on **MAR** and then on **405** to access Pablo Rodriguez's records.

2. What medications still need to be given to Pablo Rodriguez for the day shift (up to 1500)?

- Click on **Return to Nurses' Station**.
- Click on the **Drug** icon in the lower left corner of the screen.
- Use the Drug Guide to answer the next three questions.

3. How does ondansetron differ from metoclopramide in regard to antiemetic mechanism of action?

4. When ondansetron is administered by IV, it should be infused over _____ minutes.

- Click on **Return to Nurses' Station**.
- Click on **Chart** and then on **405** for Pablo Rodriguez's chart.
- Click on **Patient Education**.

5. Has any teaching been completed? In your opinion, what priority teaching should have been completed upon admission?

- Click on **Return to Nurses' Station**.
- Click on **405** at the bottom of the screen.
- Click on **Patient Care** and then on **Nurse-Client Interactions**.
- Select and view the video titled **1150: Assessment—Pain**. (*Note:* Check the virtual clock to see whether enough time has elapsed. You can use the fast-forward feature to advance the time by 2-minute intervals if the video is not yet available. Then click again on **Patient Care** and on **Nurse-Client Interactions** to refresh the screen.)

6. Why is Pablo Rodriguez not eating?

7. Is this a normal side effect of chemotherapy?

8. How would you treat this?

- Click on **Kardex** and select tab **405**. Read the outcomes.

9. What additional outcome(s) might you include for this patient?

10. What is Pablo Rodriguez's code status? How do you feel about this in relation to his diagnosis and condition? What is the nurse's professional responsibility related to the patient's code status?

10 _____

Asthma

_____

Reading Assignment: Assessment and Care of Patients with Problems of Acid-Base Balance
(Chapter 12)
Care of Patients with Noninfectious Lower Respiratory Problems
(Chapter 30)
Care of Patients with Infectious Respiratory Problems (Chapter 31)

Patient: Jacquline Catanazaro, Room 402

Goal: To utilize the nursing process to competently care for a patient with asthma.

Objectives:

1. Identify clinical manifestations of an acute asthmatic exacerbation.
2. Evaluate diagnostic tests as they relate to a patient's oxygenation status.
3. Identify medications used to treat asthma, along with their mechanism of action and therapeutic effects.
4. Prioritize nursing care for a patient with an acute exacerbation of asthma.
5. Formulate an appropriate patient education plan regarding home asthma management for a patient with identified barriers to learning.

In this lesson you will learn the essentials of caring for a patient diagnosed with asthma. You will explore the patient's history, evaluate presenting symptoms and treatment upon admission, and follow the patient's progress throughout the hospital stay. Jacquline Catanazaro is a 45-year-old female admitted with increasing respiratory distress. Her condition is further complicated by her schizophrenia. You will begin this lesson by first reviewing the general concepts of asthma as presented in your textbook.

Exercise 1

Writing Activity

30 minutes

1. Briefly describe the pathophysiology of asthma.

2. Match each description with the type of asthma it characterizes.

Description	**Asthma Type**
_____ Daytime symptoms occur less than twice a week.	a. Controlled asthma
_____ Activities are limited because of symptoms.	b. Partly controlled asthma
_____ Nighttime symptoms are present.	
_____ Peak expiratory flow (PEF) is normal.	

3. Patients with uncontrolled asthma have a minimum of how many partly controlled symptoms?
   a. 1
   b. 2
   c. 3
   d. 4

4. Fill in the correct step number in each of the blanks of this statement: The step system for medication use in asthma management includes an as-needed rapid-acting beta-2 agonist inhaler beginning with

   Step _____. An inhaled corticosteroid (ICS) is added for patients in Step _____. An oral

   glucocorticosteroid is added for patients in Step _____.

5. Match each term with its corresponding definition.

Term	Definition

_____   Forced vital capacity (FVC)

_____   Forced expiratory volume in
the first second (FEV_1)

_____   Peak expiratory flow rate (PEFR)

a. Volume of air blown out as hard and fast as possible during the first second of the most forceful exhalation after the greatest full inhalation

b. Fastest airflow rate reached at any time during exhalation

c. Volume of air exhaled from full inhalation to full exhalation

Exercise 2

Virtual Hospital Activity

40 minutes

- Sign in to work at Pacific View Regional Hospital for Period of Care 1. (*Note:* If you are already in the virtual hospital from a previous exercise, click on **Leave the Floor** and then on **Restart the Program** to get to the sign-in window.)
- From the Patient List, select Jacquline Catanazaro (Room 402).
- Click on **Go to Nurses' Station**.
- Click on **Chart** and then on **402**.
- Click on **History and Physical**.

1. What are Jacquline Catanazaro's medical diagnoses?

2. What pathologic triggers can lead to an exacerbation of asthma? (*Hint:* See Chapter 30 in your textbook.)

3. Does Jacquline Catanazaro's history identify any of these triggers?

4. What other factor(s) might be contributing to her asthma exacerbations?

- Click on **Emergency Department** and review the record.

5. What were Jacquline Catanazaro's presenting symptoms at the time of admission?

- Click on **Physician's Orders**.

6. What medical treatment is ordered in the Emergency Department? (*Hint:* See the orders for Monday at 1005.)

7. How would you evaluate the patient's response to medical treatment?

8. Review the medications ordered on Monday at 1600. Match each medication with its corresponding mechanism for each. (*Hint:* Click on **Return to Nurses' Station**; then click on the **Drug Guide** on the counter or on the **Drug** icon in the lower left corner of your screen.)

Medication

_____ Beclomethasone

_____ Albuterol

_____ Ipratropium bromide

Mechanism of Action

a. Anticholinergic that blocks the action of acetylcholine at parasympathetic sites in bronchial smooth muscle; causes bronchodilation and decreases mucosal secretions.

b. Adrenocorticosteroid used for its antiinflammatory effects. It inhibits bronchoconstriction, produces smooth muscle relaxation, and decreases mucus production.

c. Adrenergic agonist that stimulates beta$_2$-adrenergic receptors in the lungs, causing relaxation of bronchial smooth muscle; relieves bronchospasm and reduces airway resistance.

9. In what order would the nurse administer these medications? State your rationale. (*Hint:* See Chart 30-6 in the textbook, in addition to the **Drug Guide**.)

10. What new medications are ordered on Tuesday at 0800? Give a rationale for these orders. Why is the prednisone ordered to decrease by 5 mg every day?

Exercise 3

Virtual Hospital Activity

30 minutes

- Sign in to work at Pacific View Regional Hospital for Period of Care 1. (*Note:* If you are already in the virtual hospital from a previous exercise, click on **Leave the Floor** and then on **Restart the Program** to get to the sign-in window.)
- From the Patient List, select Jacquline Catanazaro (Room 402).
- Click on **Go to Nurses' Station**.
- Click on **402** at the bottom of your screen.
- Read the Initial Observations.

1. Describe your initial observations when you enter Jacquline Catanazaro's room.

- Click on **Take Vital Signs**.

2. Record Jacquline Catanazaro's vital signs below.

- Click on **Clinical Alerts**.

3. Are there any clinical alerts for Jacquline Catanazaro? If so, describe below.

4. How would you prioritize your care for the patient at this point?

• Click on **Patient Care** and then on **Physical Assessment**.

5. Perform and document a focused assessment on three priority areas based on Jacquline Catanazaro's present status. Identify these areas and record your findings below.

• Click on **Chart** and then on **402**.
• Click on **Physician's Orders**.

6. What new orders did the physician write on Monday at 0730?

• Click on **Return to Room 402**.
• Click on **Patient Care** and then on **Nurse-Client Interactions**.
• Select and view the video titled **0730: Intervention—Airway**. (*Note:* Check the virtual clock to see whether enough time has elapsed. You can use the fast-forward feature to advance the time by 2-minute intervals if the video is not yet available. Then click again on **Patient Care** and on **Nurse-Client Interactions** to refresh the screen.)

7. How does this nurse prioritize her actions? What reasons can you give for her actions?

- Click on **Clinical Alerts** and review the note for 0800. (*Note:* Check the virtual clock to see whether enough time has elapsed. You can use the fast-forward feature to advance the time by 2-minute intervals if the alert is not yet available. Then click again on **Patient Care** and on **Clinical Alerts** to refresh the screen.)

8. Give your interpretation of this alert.

- Click on **Chart** and then on **402**.
- Click on **Physician's Notes**.

9. Read the notes for Wednesday at 0800. How does the physician evaluate the patient's condition at this point?

- Click on **Physician's Orders**. Find the orders for 0800 on Wednesday.

10. Record each order below and provide a rationale for each.

Exercise 4

Virtual Hospital Activity

30 minutes

- Sign in to work at Pacific View Regional Hospital for Period of Care 2. (*Note:* If you are already in the virtual hospital from a previous exercise, click on **Leave the Floor** and then on **Restart the Program** to get to the sign-in window.)
- From the Patient List, select Jacquline Catanazaro (Room 402).
- Click on **Get Report**.

1. Briefly summarize the activity for Jacquline Catanazaro over the last 4 hours.

- Click on **Go to Nurses' Station**.
- Click on **402** at the bottom of the screen.
- Read the Initial Observations.

2. What is your initial observation of Jacquline Catanazaro for this time period?

- Click on **Take Vital Signs**.

3. How do the results of these vital signs compare with those you obtained during Period of Care 1? (*Hint:* See question 2 of Exercise 3 for those findings.)

- Click on **Patient Care** and then on **Nurse-Client Interactions**.
- Select and view the video titled **1115: Assessment—Readiness to Learn**. (*Note:* Check the virtual clock to see whether enough time has elapsed. You can use the fast-forward feature to advance the time by 2-minute intervals if the video is not yet available. Then click again on **Patient Care** and on **Nurse-Client Interactions** to refresh the screen.)

4. Describe the nurse's actions in the video. Are they appropriate? Explain.

5. What barriers to learning might be present for Jacquline Catanazaro?

- Click on **Chart** and then on **402** for Jacquline Catanazaro's chart.
- Click on **Patient Education**.

6. What are the educational goals for Jacquline Catanazaro?

7. The patient is scheduled for discharge tomorrow. Do you have any concerns? What would be your most appropriate action?

- Click on **Return to Room 402**.
- Click on **Leave the Floor**.
- Click on **Restart the Program**.
- Sign in to work at Pacific View Regional Hospital for Period of Care 3.
- From the Patient List, select Jacquline Catanazaro (Room 402).
- Click on **Go to Nurses' Station**.
- Click on **402** at the bottom of the screen.
- Click on **Patient Care** and then on **Nurse-Client Interactions**.
- Select and view the video titled **1500: Intervention—Patient Teaching**. (*Note:* Check the virtual clock to see whether enough time has elapsed. You can use the fast-forward feature to advance the time by 2-minute intervals if the video is not yet available. Then click again on **Patient Care** and on **Nurse-Client Interactions** to refresh the screen.)

8. What equipment is the nurse teaching the patient about?

9. Describe the proper use of the peak flow meter for patients.

LESSON 11

Emphysema and Pneumonia

Reading Assignment: Care of Patients with Noninfectious Lower Respiratory Problems
(Chapter 30)
Care of Patients with Infectious Respiratory Problems (Chapter 31)

Patient: Patricia Newman, Room 406

Goal: To utilize the nursing process to competently care for patients with altered oxygenation states.

Objectives:

1. Relate physical assessment findings with pathophysiologic changes of the lower respiratory tract.
2. Prioritize nursing care for a patient with altered oxygenation.
3. Evaluate laboratory results relative to the diagnosis of pneumonia and emphysema.
4. Describe pharmacologic interventions related to altered oxygenation states.
5. Identify appropriate nursing interventions for a patient admitted with pneumonia and emphysema.
6. Identify appropriate discharge teaching needs for a patient with altered oxygenation.

In this lesson you will learn the essentials of caring for a patient diagnosed with pneumonia and emphysema. You will explore the patient's history, evaluate presenting symptoms and treatment upon admission, and assess the patient's progress throughout the hospital stay. Patricia Newman is a 61-year-old female admitted with pneumonia and a history of emphysema. You will begin this lesson by first reviewing the general concepts of altered oxygenation states as presented in your textbook.

Exercise 1

Writing Activity

20 minutes

1. To which category of lung diseases does emphysema belong?

2. Briefly describe the pathophysiology of emphysema.

3. Briefly describe the pathophysiology of pneumonia.

4. Which are risk factors for community-acquired pneumonia? Select all that apply.

_____ Older adult

_____ History of chronic lung disease

_____ Uses tobacco products

_____ Uses alcohol

_____ Poor nutritional status

_____ Recent exposure to influenza infection

_____ Has not received pneumococcal vaccination in the past 5 years

5. When caring for a patient with pneumonia, empyema may result. What does this entail?
   a. The lung collapses.
   b. There is a solidification in one of the lung's lobes.
   c. Bacteria has infiltrated the blood stream.
   d. There is a collection of pus in the pleural cavity.

6. Which is the most common cause of bacterial pneumonia?
    a. *Staphylococcus*
    b. *Streptococcus*
    c. *Pneumococcus*
    d. *Meningococcus*

Exercise 2

Virtual Hospital Activity

45 minutes

- Sign in to work at Pacific View Regional Hospital for Period of Care 1. (*Note:* If you are already in the virtual hospital from a previous exercise, click on **Leave the Floor** and then on **Restart the Program** to get to the sign-in window.)
- From the Patient List, select Patricia Newman (Room 406).
- Click on **Get Report**.

1. What questions would you ask the outgoing nurses to obtain needed information that was not identified in the report?

2. Match the clinical manifestations identified in the report with the pathophysiologic basis of each manifestation.

Clinical Manifestation	Pathophysiologic Basis
_____ Dyspnea	a. Release of pyrogens by phagocytes, which triggers hypothalamus
_____ Fever	b. Fluid from pulmonary capillaries and RBCs invades alveoli
_____ Cough	c. Fluid accumulation triggers receptors in trachea, bronchi, and bronchioles
_____ Yellow sputum	d. Increased work of breathing, pain, and anxiety

- Click on **Go to Nurses' Station**.
- Click on **Chart** and then on **406**.
- Click on **History and Physical**.

3. What risk factors for community-acquired pneumonia does Patricia Newman have?

- Click on **Nursing Admission**.

4. What other risk factor for community-acquired pneumonia is documented on this form?

- Click on **Return to Nurses' Station**.
- Click on **406** at the bottom of your screen.
- Read the Initial Observations.
- Click on **Take Vital Signs**.

5. What should be your priority nursing assessment/intervention(s) based on your initial observation of Patricia Newman?

- Click on **Patient Care** and then on **Physical Assessment**.

6. Perform a focused assessment based on Patricia Newman's admitting diagnosis by clicking on the body categories (yellow buttons) and subcategories (green buttons). Record your findings for respiratory, cardiovascular, and mental status assessments below. How has her condition changed since report?

Respiratory

Cardiovascular

Mental Status

- Click on **Patient Care** and then on **Nurse-Client Interactions**.
- Select and view the video titled **0730: Prioritizing Interventions**. (*Note:* Check the virtual clock to see whether enough time has elapsed. You can use the fast-forward feature to advance the time by 2-minute intervals if the video is not yet available. Then click again on **Patient Care** and on **Nurse-Client Interactions** to refresh the screen.)

7. Evaluate the nurse's actions based on the patient's current status. How does this nurse's action differ from your plan of care you outlined in question 5 of this exercise?

8. What nursing interventions might be done to alleviate the patient's anxiety?

- Click on **Chart** and then on **406** for Patricia Newman's chart.
- Click on **Laboratory Reports**.

9. Identify any abnormal laboratory results and describe how they correlate with Patricia Newman's diagnosis of pneumonia.

- Click on **Return to Room 406**.
- Click on **Drug Guide** in the lower left-hand corner to access the Drug Guide.

10. What is the desired therapeutic effect of ipratropium bromide? How could the nurse assess whether the desired effect was achieved?

11. What is the desired therapeutic effect of cefotetan? How could the nurse assess whether the desired effect was achieved?

12. What is the rationale for administration of IV fluids related to pneumonia?

- Click on **Return to Room 406**.
- Click on **Medication Room**.
- Click on **MAR** to determine medications that Patricia Newman is ordered to receive at 0800 and any prn medications you may want to administer. (*Note:* You may click on **Review MAR** at any time to verify correct medication order. You must click on the correct room number within the MAR. Remember to look at the patient name on the MAR to make sure you have the correct patient's record. Click on **Return to Medication Room** after reviewing the correct MAR.)
- Click on **Unit Dosage**; then click on drawer **406**.
- Select the medication(s) you plan to administer. After each medication you select, click on **Put Medication on Tray**. When you are finished, click on **Close Drawer**.
- Click on **View Medication Room**.
- Click on **IV Storage**. From the close-up view, click on the drawer labeled **Large Volume**.
- Select the medication(s) you plan to administer, put medication(s) on tray, and close bin.
- Click on **View Medication Room**.
- Click on **Preparation**. Select the correct medication to administer; click on **Prepare** and on **Next**.
- Wait for the Preparation Wizard to appear; then provide any information requested.
- Choose the correct patient to administer this medication to and click on **Finish**.
- Repeat the above three steps until all medications that you want to administer are prepared.
- You can click on **Review Your Medications** and then on **Return to Medication Room** when ready. From the Medication Room, you may go directly to Patricia Newman's room by clicking on **406** at the bottom of the screen.
- Administer the medication, utilizing the six rights of medication administration. After you have collected the appropriate assessment data and are ready for administration, click on **Patient Care** and then on **Medication Administration**. Verify that the correct patient and medication(s) appear in the left-hand window. Then click the down arrow next to Select. From the drop-down menu, select **Administer** and complete the Administration Wizard by providing any information requested. When the Wizard stops asking for information, click on **Administer to Patient**. Specify **Yes** when asked whether this administration should be recorded in the MAR. Finally, click on **Finish**.

Now let's see how you did!

- Click on **Leave the Floor** at the bottom of your screen. From the Floor Menu, select **Look at Your Preceptor's Evaluation**. Then click on **Medication Scorecard**.

13. Note below whether or not you correctly administered the appropriate medications. If not, why do you think you were incorrect? According to Table C in this scorecard, what are the appropriate resources that should be used and important assessments that should be completed before administering these medications? Did you use these resources and perform these assessments correctly?

Exercise 3

Virtual Hospital Activity

40 minutes

- Sign in to work at Pacific View Regional Hospital for Period of Care 2. (*Note:* If you are already in the virtual hospital from a previous exercise, click on **Leave the Floor** and then on **Restart the Program** to get to the sign-in window.)
- From the Patient List, select Patricia Newman (Room 406).
- Click on **Go to Nurses' Station**.
- Click on **Chart** and then on **406**.
- Click on **History and Physical**.

1. How long has Patricia Newman been diagnosed with emphysema?

2. What clinical manifestations documented on the History and Physical can be attributed to emphysema?

- Click on **Diagnostic Reports**.

3. What findings on the chest x-ray are consistent with the diagnosis of emphysema?

4. What is the relationship between the patient's admitting diagnosis (pneumonia) and her underlying chronic condition (emphysema)?

- Click on **Patient Education**.

5. What is educational goal 3 for Patricia Newman?

6. Explain how you would teach the patient to achieve goal 3.

7. What is educational goal 4 for Patricia Newman?

8. What do you think Patricia Newman's special dietary needs are? Explain your answer.

9. What is educational goal 6 for Patricia Newman?

10. What is the rationale for your answer to the previous question? How would you teach this technique to Patricia Newman?

11. Because Patricia Newman's emphysema puts her at high risk for pulmonary infections, what would you teach her to do to help prevent further episodes of pneumonia? (*Hint:* See Chart 31-3 of your textbook.)

- Click on **Return to Nurses' Station**.
- Click on **406**.
- Click on **Patient Care** and then on **Nurse-Client Interactions**.
- Select and view the video titled **1100: Care Coordination**. (*Note:* Check the virtual clock to see whether enough time has elapsed. You can use the fast-forward feature to advance the time by 2-minute intervals if the video is not yet available. Then click again on **Patient Care** and on **Nurse-Client Interactions** to refresh the screen.)

12. Discuss the three disciplines for which representatives are set to visit Patricia Newman today, including the role of each discipline in helping meet her health care needs.

LESSON 12

Pulmonary Embolism

Reading Assignment: Care of Critically Ill Patients with Respiratory Problems (Chapter 32)

Patient: Clarence Hughes, Room 404

Goal: To utilize the nursing process to competently care for patients with a critically altered oxygenation state.

Objectives:

1. Identify clinical manifestations of pulmonary embolism.
2. Prioritize nursing care for a patient with acute onset of respiratory distress and chest pain.
3. Describe diagnostic testing relative to the diagnosis of pulmonary embolism.
4. Describe pharmacologic therapy for a patient with a pulmonary embolism.
5. Accurately calculate the correct dosage of heparin for a patient using a sliding scale.
6. Identify disease management issues regarding the care of a patient with a pulmonary embolism.

In this lesson you will learn the essentials of caring for a patient diagnosed with an acute pulmonary embolism. You will explore the patient's history, evaluate presenting symptoms and treatment, provide appropriate nursing interventions, and assess the patient's progress throughout the clinical day. Clarence Hughes is a 73-year-old male admitted for an elective left knee arthroplasty.

Exercise 1

Writing Activity

5 minutes

1. Describe the pathophysiology of pulmonary embolism.

2. List common sources of pulmonary emboli.

3. Which are factors for the development of a pulmonary embolism? Select all that apply.

_____   Advancing age

_____   Heredity

_____   Obesity

_____   Immobility

_____   Recent surgery

_____   Central venous catheters

Exercise 2

Virtual Hospital Activity

30 minutes

- Sign in to work at Pacific View Regional Hospital for Period of Care 2. (*Note:* If you are already in the virtual hospital from a previous exercise, click on **Leave the Floor** and then on **Restart the Program** to get to the sign-in window.)
- From the Patient List, select Clarence Hughes (Room 404).
- Click on **Get Report**.
- Click on **Go to Nurses' Station**.
- Click on **404** at the bottom of your screen.

1. What is your initial observation as you enter the patient's room?

2. What should your priority actions be at this point?

- Click on **Patient Care** and then on **Nurse-Client Interactions**.
- Select and view the video titled **1115: Interventions—Airway**. (*Note:* Check the virtual clock to see whether enough time has elapsed. You can use the fast-forward feature to advance the time by 2-minute intervals if the video is not yet available. Then click again on **Patient Care** and on **Nurse-Client Interactions** to refresh the screen.)

3. Review the nurse's actions. Was it appropriate for her to leave Clarence Hughes to get the oxygen? Why or why not? If not, what else could she have done?

4. What classic signs and symptoms of pulmonary embolism is Clarence Hughes displaying?

5. Suspecting a pulmonary embolus, for what other clinical manifestations would you assess Clarence Hughes? (*Hint:* See Chapter 32 in your textbook.)

- Click on **Chart** and then on **404** for Clarence Hughes' chart.
- Click on **History and Physical**.

6. Based on the patient's history and current reason for hospitalization, what risk factors for deep vein thrombosis (DVT) and resultant pulmonary embolism does Clarence Hughes have?

• Click on **Physician's Orders**.

7. Look at the orders dated Wednesday at 1120. Document these orders below and provide a rationale for each order.

• Click on **Return to Room 404**.
• Click on **Patient Care** and then on **Nurse-Client Interactions**.
• Select and view the video titled **1135: Change in Patient Condition**. (*Note:* Check the virtual clock to see whether enough time has elapsed. You can use the fast-forward feature to advance the time by 2-minute intervals if the video is not yet available. Then click again on **Patient Care** and on **Nurse-Client Interactions** to refresh the screen.)

8. As the nurse is explaining care to the family, she states that a transporter will be coming to take Clarence Hughes for a ventilation-perfusion scan. Would you send this patient down to radiology with just the transporter? Why or why not?

Exercise 3

Virtual Hospital Activity

30 minutes

- Sign in to work at Pacific View Regional Hospital for Period of Care 3. (*Note:* If you are already in the virtual hospital from a previous exercise, click on **Leave the Floor** and then on **Restart the Program** to get to the sign-in window.)
- From the Patient List, select Clarence Hughes (Room 404).
- Click on **Go to Nurses' Station**.
- Click on **Chart** and then on **404** for Clarence Hughes' chart.
- Select and review the **Laboratory Reports** and **Diagnostic Reports**.

1. Below, document the results of the ordered diagnostic and laboratory testing. Please note that the laboratory results are reported for Wednesday at 1130.

2. Based on the above results, what would you conclude to be the cause of Clarence Hughes' acute respiratory distress?

- Click on **Physician's Orders**.

3. What orders were written to treat Clarence Hughes' pulmonary embolism?

4. What laboratory test will be used to titrate the heparin infusion? What are the normal values for this test?

5. What is the desired therapeutic level for this laboratory test?

- Click on **Return to Nurses' Station**.
- Click on **MAR** and then on **404** for Clarence Hughes' record.

6. How many mL of heparin would you administer for the bolus dose if the medication on hand is heparin 5000 units/mL?

7. If you were the nurse starting the heparin infusion, at what rate would you set the IV pump to infuse this medication?

- Click on **Return to Nurses' Station**.
- Click on **Chart** and then on **404** for Clarence Hughes' record.
- Click on **Laboratory Reports**.

8. What were the results of the PTT and INR at 1300 today? Why were these tests ordered prior to starting the heparin?

- Click on **Return to Nurses' Station**.
- Click on **404** to enter Clarence Hughes' room.
- Click on **Patient Care** and then on **Nurse-Client Interactions**.
- Select and view the video titled **1510: Disease Management**. (*Note:* Check the virtual clock to see whether enough time has elapsed. You can use the fast-forward feature to advance the time by 2-minute intervals if the video is not yet available. Then click again on **Patient Care** and on **Nurse-Client Interactions** to refresh the screen.)

9. When the patient's son asks the nurse whether the pulmonary embolism will delay his father's discharge, the nurse states that the heparin takes 2 days to stabilize. Does this mean that the patient will be discharged on heparin? If not, what medication will be used to minimize clot formation? Explain why the patient is not started on this medication rather than heparin.

10. What lab test(s) will be used to monitor the therapeutic effect of warfarin (Coumadin)? What is the therapeutic range for these tests?

11. For what possible complications would you monitor Clarence Hughes related to the pulmonary embolism?

Exercise 4

Virtual Hospital Activity

20 minutes

- Sign in to work at Pacific View Regional Hospital for Period of Care 4. (*Note:* If you are already in the virtual hospital from a previous exercise, click on **Leave the Floor** and then on **Restart the Program** to get to the sign-in window.)
- Click on **Chart** and then on **404** for Clarence Hughes' chart. (*Remember:* You are not able to visit patients or administer medications during Period of Care 4. You are able to review patient records only.)
- Click on **Laboratory Reports**.

1. What is the PTT result for 1900?

- Click on **Return to Nurses' Station**.
- Click on **MAR** and then on **404** for Clarence Hughes' record.
- Click on **Physician's Orders**.

2. What would you do now with the heparin infusion? Calculate the correct infusion rate and document below.

- Click on **Return to Nurses' Station**.
- Click on **Kardex** and then on **404** for Clarence Hughes' record.

3. Are there any additional outcomes that should be added based on the patient's current setback? If so, list these outcomes.

4. If the heparin is not effective in treating Clarence Hughes and his condition worsens, what other pharmacologic treatment might be helpful? Explain.

5. Describe appropriate nursing interventions to prevent injury for Clarence Hughes while he is receiving anticoagulant and/or fibrinolytic therapy.

6. If Clarence Hughes' condition deteriorates, what surgical treatment might be needed? Explain.

7. If this patient develops another pulmonary embolus, what further treatment might the physician consider to prevent the problem from recurring in the future? Explain.

Atrial Fibrillation

Reading Assignment: Assessment and Care of Patients with Problems of Fluid and
Electrolyte Balance (Chapter 11)
Care of Patients with Dysrhythmias (Chapter 34)

Patient: Piya Jordan, Room 403

Goal: To utilize the nursing process to competently care for patients with atrial fibrillation.

Objectives:

1. Describe telemetry rhythm strip characteristics of atrial fibrillation.
2. Identify potential etiologies of atrial fibrillation for an assigned patient.
3. Assess a patient for clinical manifestations of atrial fibrillation.
4. Identify potential complications of atrial fibrillation.
5. Perform appropriate assessments before administering pharmacologic therapy for atrial fibrillation.
6. Accurately administer IV digoxin.
7. Discuss the use of anticoagulation therapy for a patient with atrial fibrillation.
8. Develop appropriate educational outcomes for a patient with a history of atrial fibrillation.

In this lesson you will learn the essentials of caring for a patient with a cardiac dysrhythmia. You will
explore the patient's history, evaluate presenting symptoms and treatment, provide appropriate nursing
interventions, and plan appropriate patient educational outcomes related to the dysrhythmia. Piya Jordan
is a 68-year-old female admitted with nausea, vomiting, and abdominal pain.

Exercise 1

Writing Activity

20 minutes

1. Describe the normal conduction system of the heart.

2. What is "atrial kick"? Why is this important?

3. Identify the cardiac event represented by each of the waves and measured intervals:

   a. P wave

   b. PR interval

   c. QRS complex

   d. T wave

   e. U wave

   f. QT interval

4. Identify and describe the eight steps of electrocardiogram (ECG) analysis.

  (1)

  (2)

  (3)

  (4)

  (5)

  (6)

  (7)

  (8)

Exercise 2

Virtual Hospital Activity

35 minutes

- Sign in to work at Pacific View Regional Hospital for Period of Care 1. (*Note:* If you are already in the virtual hospital from a previous exercise, click on **Leave the Floor** and then on **Restart the Program** to get to the sign-in window.)
- From the Patient List, select Piya Jordan (Room 403).
- Click on **Go to Nurses' Station**.
- Click on **403** at the bottom of your screen. Read the Initial Observations.

  1. What information regarding Piya Jordan's cardiovascular status is obtained on initial observation?

2. What is telemetry monitoring?

3. During atrial fibrillation the atria depolarize in a disorganized manner at a rate of _____

   to _____ times per minute.

4. Describe the rhythm strip you would expect to see on Piya Jordan's monitor.

5. How does this differ from normal sinus rhythm?

• Click on **Take Vital Signs**.

6. Record Piya Jordan's heart rate below and state whether the rhythm is controlled
   (ventricular rate less than 100) or uncontrolled (ventricular rate greater than 100) atrial
   fibrillation.

7. For what clinical manifestations consistent with atrial fibrillation should Piya Jordan be assessed?
   Select all that apply. (*Hint:* See Chapter 34 in your textbook.)

   _____ Fatigue

   _____ Restlessness

   _____ Lethargy

   _____ Weakness

   _____ Shortness of breath

   _____ Dizziness

   _____ Palpitations

   _____ Hypertension

   _____ Syncope

   _____ Chest discomfort

- Click on **Patient Care** and then on **Physical Assessment**.
- Complete a general assessment of Piya Jordan by clicking on the body system categories (yellow buttons) and subcategories (green buttons).

8. Does Piya Jordan present with any symptoms that are associated with atrial fibrillation? If not, how can you explain that?

9. If Piya Jordan's heart rate increases, how might the atrial fibrillation affect her blood pressure? Describe the underlying physiology. (*Hint:* Think about normal atrial kick.)

- Click on **Chart** and then on **403**.
- Click on **Diagnostic Reports**.

10. Did Piya Jordan have a 12-lead ECG done? If yes, what was the rhythm? If not, do you think it should have been done? Why or why not?

11. For what potential complications related to atrial fibrillation should you monitor Piya Jordan? Describe appropriate nursing assessments related to each complication. (*Hint:* See Chapter 34 in your textbook.)

Exercise 3

Virtual Hospital Activity

45 minutes

- Sign in to work at Pacific View Regional Hospital for Period of Care 1. (*Note:* If you are already in the virtual hospital from a previous exercise, click on **Leave the Floor** and then on **Restart the Program** to get to the sign-in window.)
- From the Patient List, select Piya Jordan (Room 403).
- Click on **Go to Nurses' Station**.
- Click on **MAR** and then on tab **403**.

1. What medication is prescribed to treat Piya Jordan's atrial fibrillation? Describe the pharmacodynamics of this medication as related to atrial fibrillation. (*Hint:* You may need to consult the Drug Guide.)

2. Why did the physician order a digoxin level when the patient first presented to the Emergency Department? (*Hint:* Review the patient's presenting symptoms as well as the Drug Guide.)

- Click on **Return to Nurses' Station**.
- Click on **Chart** and then on **403**.
- Click on **Laboratory Reports**.

3. Piya Jordan's digoxin level in the Emergency Department was _____ ng/mL.

4. The digoxin level you recorded in question 3 is considered:
    a. subtherapeutic.
    b. therapeutic.
    c. toxic.

5. For what symptoms of digoxin toxicity would you monitor Piya Jordan? Select all that apply.

_____   Tachycardia

_____   Visual disturbances

_____   Headache

_____   Nausea

_____   Constipation

_____   Anorexia

_____   Fatigue

_____   Labile emotions

_____   Facial pain

_____   Personality changes

6. Piya Jordan's potassium level in the Emergency Department was _____ mEq/L.

7. How does this relate to possible digoxin toxicity? (*Hint:* See Chapter 11 in your textbook.)

- Click on **History and Physical**.

8. What other medication was Piya Jordan prescribed related to atrial fibrillation before this admission? Explain the rationale for this medication. (*Hint:* Think of potential serious complications of atrial fibrillation.)

- Click on **Physician's Orders**.

9. What two items, ordered on Tuesday at 0130 and at 0800, did the physician prescribe preoperatively to reverse Piya Jordan's anticoagulation? How would you know whether they were effective? Explain.

10. What medication was ordered postoperatively on Wednesday at 0730 to prevent clot formation?

- Click on **Nursing Admission**.

11. What knowledge (or lack of knowledge) does Piya Jordan verbalize regarding her history of atrial fibrillation? (*Hint:* Look at the Health Promotion section.)

- Click on **Patient Education**.

12. What might you add to these outcomes based on your answer to question 11?

13. What surgical treatment options may be used for patients with recurrent or sustained atrial fibrillation?

- Click on **Return to Nurses' Station**.
- Click on **Medication Room**.
- Click on **MAR** to determine medications that Piya Jordan is ordered to receive at 0800. (*Note:* You may click on **Review MAR** at any time to verify correct medication order. You must click on the room number tab within the MAR. Remember to look at the patient name on the MAR to make sure you have the correct patient's record. Click on **Return to Medication Room** after reviewing the correct MAR.)
- Based on your care for Piya Jordan, access the various storage areas of the Medication Room to obtain the necessary medications you need to administer.
- For each area you access, first select the medication you plan to administer and then click on **Put Medication on Tray**. When finished with a storage area, click on **Close Drawer**.
- Click on **View Medication Room**.
- Click on **Preparation** and choose the correct medication to administer. Click on **Prepare**.
- Wait for the Preparation Wizard to appear; then provide any information requested.
- Click on **Next** and choose the correct patient to administer the medication to. Click on **Finish**.

- Repeat the above three steps until all medications that you want to administer are prepared.
- You can click on **Review Your Medications** and then on **Return to Medication Room** when you are ready. Once you are back in the Medication Room, you may go directly to Piya Jordan's room by clicking on **403** at the bottom of the screen.
- Administer the medication, utilizing the six rights of medication administration. After you have collected the appropriate assessment data and are ready for administration, click on **Patient Care** and then on **Medication Administration**. Verify that the correct patient and medication(s) appear in the left-hand window. Then click the down arrow next to Select. From the drop-down menu, select **Administer** and complete the Administration Wizard by providing any information requested. When the Wizard stops asking for information, click **Administer to Patient**. Specify **Yes** when asked whether this administration should be recorded in the MAR. Finally, click on **Finish**.

14. You should administer the IV digoxin over _____ minutes.

15. What should you have assessed before administering digoxin to Piya Jordan today?

Now let's see how you did!

- Click on **Leave the Floor** at the bottom of your screen. From the Floor Menu, click on **Look at Your Preceptor's Evaluation**.
- Click on **Medication Scorecard**.

16. Note below whether or not you correctly administered the appropriate medication(s). If not, why do you think you were incorrect? According to Table C in this scorecard, what resources should be used and what important assessments should be completed before administering the medication(s)? Did you utilize these resources and perform these assessments correctly?

Hypertension

Reading Assignment: Care of Patients with Vascular Problems (Chapter 36)

Patients: Harry George, Room 401
Patricia Newman, Room 406

Goal: To utilize the nursing process to competently care for patients with hypertension.

Objectives:

1. Describe the blood pressure (BP) treatment goals.
2. Identify the presence of risk factors for hypertension in assigned patients.
3. Discuss pharmacologic therapies available to treat hypertension.
4. Perform appropriate assessments before administering pharmacologic therapy for hypertension.
5. Develop an extensive educational plan for patients with hypertension.

In this lesson you will learn the essentials of caring for a patient with hypertension. You will explore the patient's history, evaluate presenting symptoms and treatment, provide appropriate nursing interventions, and plan an appropriate patient educational plan related to the hypertension. Patricia Newman is a 61-year-old female admitted with pneumonia and a history of emphysema. Harry George is a 54-year-old male admitted with infection and swelling of the left foot.

Exercise 1

Writing Activity

15 minutes

1. Match each age group with the appropriate goal of hypertension management.

Age Group	Goal
_____ Patients over the age of 60 years	a. BP less than 140/90
_____ Patients younger than 60 years	b. BP less than 150/90
_____ Patients over the age of 18 years, with chronic kidney disease	

2. Define the following terms:

   a. Malignant hypertension

   b. Secondary hypertension

   c. Orthostatic hypotension

3. Match each type of hypertension with its potential causes.

Potential Cause	Type of Hypertension
_____ Pregnancy	a. Primary
_____ Brain tumors	b. Secondary
_____ Excessive caffeine intake	
_____ Excessive sodium intake	
_____ Obesity	
_____ Inactivity	
_____ Kidney disease	

Exercise 2

Virtual Hospital Activity

45 minutes

- Sign in to work at Pacific View Regional Hospital for Period of Care 1. (*Note:* If you are already in the virtual hospital from a previous exercise, click on **Leave the Floor** and then on **Restart the Program** to get to the sign-in window.)
- From the Patient List, select Patricia Newman (Room 406).
- Click on **Go to Nurses' Station**.
- Click on **Chart** and then on **406**.
- Click on **History and Physical**.

1. How long has Patricia Newman been diagnosed with hypertension?

- Click on **Nursing Admission**.

2. What recorded factors increase her risk for hypertension?

- Click on **Physician's Orders**.

3. List the two medications ordered to treat Patricia Newman's hypertension. For each medication, identify the drug classification and its mechanism of action.

4. What baseline nursing assessments should be completed before administering each of the medications you identified in question 3?

5. For what common side effects will the nurse need to monitor the patient?

- Click on **Return to Nurses' Station**.
- Click on **EPR** and on **Login**.
- Choose **406** from the Patient drop-down menu and **Vital Signs** from the Category drop-down menu.

6. What are Patricia Newman's documented BP measurements since admission?

7. Is her prescribed antihypertensive medication currently effective? Explain.

8. Considering Patricia Newman's risk factors, what might be contributing to her currently elevated BP?

- Click on **Return to Nurses' Station**.
- Click on **Chart** and then on **406**.
- Click on **History and Physical**.

9. What indicates that Patricia Newman is in need of further teaching regarding hypertension? (*Hint:* Read the Review of Systems.)

10. What additional educational goals would be appropriate for this patient?

11. Identify lifestyle modifications that might help lower a patient's blood pressure.

- Click on **Nursing Admission**.

12. Was Patricia Newman following any of the above lifestyle modifications to lower her BP at home? Explain.

- Click on **Physician's Orders**.

13. Identify any of the modifications you addressed in question 11 that were ordered for Patricia Newman during this hospital stay.

14. As the nurse caring for Patricia Newman, what do you think would be your professional responsibility related to your findings for questions 12 and 13?

15. When planning Patricia Newman's diet, what is the recommended limit for her sodium intake?
    a. 1200 mg/day
    b. 1500 mg/day
    c. 2000 mg/day
    d. 2400 mg/day

Exercise 3

Virtual Hospital Activity

40 minutes

- Sign in to work at Pacific View Regional Hospital for Period of Care 1. (*Note:* If you are already in the virtual hospital from a previous exercise, click on **Leave the Floor** and then on **Restart the Program** to get to the sign-in window.)
- From the Patient List, select Harry George (Room 401).
- Click on **Go to Nurses' Station**.
- Click on **Chart** and then on **401**.
- Click on **History and Physical**.

1. _____ Harry George has a history of hypertension. (True or False)

2. Does he have any risk factors for hypertension? If yes, please identify.

- Click on **Return to Nurses' Station**.
- Click on **EPR** and then on **Login**.
- Choose **401** from the Patient drop-down menu and **Vital Signs** from the Category drop-down menu.

3. Document Harry George's blood pressures for the times specified below.

   Tues 0305

   Tues 0705

   Tues 1105

   Tues 1505

   Tues 1905

   Tues 2305

   Wed 0305

   Wed 0705

4. Based on the readings that you recorded in question 3, Harry George has what type of hypertension?
   a. Primary
   b. Secondary
   c. Malignant

5. What potential complications should you assess for pertaining to untreated hypertension?

- Click on **Return to Nurses' Station**.
- Click on **Chart** and then on **401**.
- Click on **Physician's Orders**.

6. The following diagnostic tests were ordered by the physician. Although these tests may have been ordered for various purposes, they might specifically help to identify target organ disease. Describe how each of the listed tests might be helpful.

Chest x-ray

BUN

Creatinine

Urinalysis

- Click on **Diagnostic Reports**.

7. Record the results of the chest x-ray. Do the results suggest the presence of target organ disease?

- Click on **Laboratory Reports.**

8. Find the laboratory results for BUN, creatinine, and urinalysis and record these below. Indicate whether these results suggest the presence of target organ disease.

9. Match each of the drugs used to manage hypertension with the appropriate mechanism of action.

Drug	Mechanism of Action
_____ Thiazide diuretics	a. Block the action of angiotensin-converting enzyme; prevent conversion of angiotensin I to angiotensin II, a potent vasoconstrictor; decrease vessel constriction
_____ Loop diuretics	
_____ Potassium-sparing diuretics	b. Inhibit reabsorption of sodium in exchange for potassium in the distal tubule; retain potassium
_____ Calcium channel blockers	c. Interfere with the transmembrane flux of calcium ions, resulting in vasodilation
_____ Angiotensin-converting enzyme (ACE) inhibitors	d. Prevent sodium and water reabsorption in the distal tubules; cause potassium excretion
_____ Angiotensin II receptor blockers (ARBs)	e. Selectively block the binding of angiotensin II to its receptor in the vascular and adrenal tissues
	f. Decrease sodium reabsorption in the ascending loop of Henle; cause sodium and potassium excretion

10. Which symptoms, if displayed by Harry George, would be consistent with a hypertensive crisis? Select all that apply.

_____   Excessive nausea

_____   Severe headache

_____   Blurred vision

_____   Anxiety

_____   Nose bleeds

11. How would you respond if a hypertensive crisis occurred? (*Hint:* See Chapter 36 in your textbook.)

Blood Transfusions

Reading Assignment: Care of Patients with Hematologic Problems (Chapter 40)

Patient: Piya Jordan, Room 403

Goal: To utilize the nursing process to competently care for patients receiving various blood products.

Objectives:

1. Describe the ABO and Rh antigen systems.
2. Identify the correct type blood to administer to a specific patient.
3. Describe appropriate nursing responsibilities related to blood product administration.
4. Evaluate vital sign assessments related to potential blood transfusion reactions.
5. Describe appropriate assessment parameters when monitoring for various types of transfusion reactions.

In this lesson you will learn the essentials of caring for a patient receiving blood and blood product transfusions. You will describe pretransfusion responsibilities, identify administration specifics, and evaluate the patient during and after each transfusion. Piya Jordan is a 68-year-old female admitted with nausea, vomiting, and abdominal pain.

Exercise 1

Writing Activity

10 minutes

1. Describe the ABO antigen system.

2. Describe the Rh antigen system.

3. For each blood type listed below, identify the type(s) of blood a patient with that type can receive. (*Hint:* See Table 40-7 in your textbook.)

A+

A–

B+

B–

O+

O–

AB+

AB–

Exercise 2

Virtual Hospital Activity

30 minutes

- Sign in to work at Pacific View Regional Hospital for Period of Care 1. (*Note:* If you are already in the virtual hospital from a previous exercise, click on **Leave the Floor** and then on **Restart the Program** to get to the sign-in window.)
- From the Patient List, select Piya Jordan (Room 403).
- Click on **Go to Nurses' Station.**
- Click on **Chart** and then on **403**.
- Click on **Laboratory Reports**.

1. Document the results of Piya Jordan's hematology tests by filling in the blanks below.

   On Monday at 2200, the hemoglobin was _____ g/dL and the hematocrit was _____%.

   On Tuesday at 0630, the hemoglobin was _____ g/dL and the hematocrit was _____%.

   On Wednesday at 0630, the hemoglobin was _____ g/dL and the hematocrit was _____%.

- Click on **Return to Nurses' Station**.
- Click on **EPR**; then click on **Login**.
- Select **403** from the Patient drop-down menu and **Intake and Output** from the Category drop-down menu. Scroll to Tuesday at 1900.

2. Why do you think Piya Jordan's Hgb and Hct are lower on Wednesday?

- Click on **Return to Nurses' Station**.
- Click on **Chart** and then on **403**.
- Click on **Physician's Orders**.

3. What was ordered to correct this? Is this appropriate related to Piya Jordan's level of hemoglobin? Explain why or why not.

- Click on **Return to Nurses' Station**.
- Click on **403** at the bottom of the screen.
- Click on **Patient Care** and then on **Nurse-Client Interactions**.
- Select and view the video titled **0735: Pain—Adverse Drug Event**. (*Note:* Check the virtual clock to see whether enough time has elapsed. You can use the fast-forward feature to advance the time by 2-minute intervals if the video is not yet available. Then click again on **Patient Care** and on **Nurse-Client Interactions** to refresh the screen.)

4. What does the nurse state she will do to prepare Piya Jordan for a blood transfusion?

5. When planning to start an IV for Piya Jordan's blood transfusion, what gauge needle should be utilized?
   a. 14-gauge
   b. 20-gauge
   c. 22-gauge
   d. 26-gauge

6. The correct IV fluid to use with a blood transfusion is:
   a. normal saline.
   b. dextrose in 5% lactated Ringer's solution.
   c. lactated Ringer's solution.
   d. 0.45% normal saline.

7. Using Ringer's lactate (lactated Ringer's) or dextrose IV solution may result in which two possible consequences?

8. What other pretransfusion responsibilities would you complete? (*Hint:* See Chapter 40 in your textbook.)

- Click on **Chart** and then on **403**.
- Click on **Laboratory Reports**.

9. What day and time was the type and cross-match completed? According to your textbook, is this laboratory result acceptable for blood being transfused today?

Exercise 3

Virtual Hospital Activity

30 minutes

- Sign in to work at Pacific View Regional Hospital for Period of Care 2. (*Note:* If you are already in the virtual hospital from a previous exercise, click on **Leave the Floor** and then on **Restart the Program** to get to the sign-in window.)
- From the Patient List, select Piya Jordan (Room 403).
- Click on **Go to Nurses' Station**.
- Click on **403** to enter Piya Jordan's room.
- Click on **Patient Care** and then on **Nurse-Client Interactions**.
- Select and view the video titled **1115: Interventions—Nausea, Blood**. (*Note:* Check the virtual clock to see whether enough time has elapsed. You can use the fast-forward feature to advance the time by 2-minute intervals if the video is not yet available. Then click again on **Patient Care** and on **Nurse-Client Interactions** to refresh the screen.)

1. Piya Jordan's daughter verbalizes concern regarding the safety of the blood transfusion. How did the nurse respond to this?

2. During the video, the nurse states that the blood has just arrived. How soon should the nurse begin the transfusion?

- Click on **Chart** and then on **403**.
- Click on **Laboratory Reports**.

3. What is Piya Jordan's blood type?

4. What type of blood may she receive safely?

5. Describe the nurse's responsibilities during the transfusion.

6. How fast would you transfuse this unit of blood? Give your rationale.

7. What assessments should be completed on Piya Jordan during the transfusion?

8. What would you document regarding this blood transfusion?

Exercise 4

Virtual Hospital Activity

40 minutes

- Sign in to work at Pacific View Regional Hospital for Period of Care 4. (*Note:* If you are already in the virtual hospital from a previous exercise, click on **Leave the Floor** and then on **Restart the Program** to get to the sign-in window.)
- Click on **EPR** and then on **Login**. (*Remember:* You are not able to visit patients or administer medications during Period of Care 4. You are only able to review patient records.)
- Select **403** from the Patient drop-down menu and **Vital Signs** from the Category drop-down menu.

1. Record Piya Jordan's vital signs (temperature, heart rate, blood pressure, and respiratory rate) during the transfusion of each of the two units of blood. The first unit vitals start on Wednesday at 1130 and end at 1400. The second unit vitals start on Wednesday at 1415 and end at 1530.

   Unit 1

   Wed 1130:

   Wed 1145:

   Wed 1200:

   Wed 1215:

   Wed 1315:

   Wed 1400:

   Unit 2

   Wed 1415:

   Wed 1430:

   Wed 1445:

   Wed 1500:

   Wed 1515:

   Wed 1530:

2. According to the above vital sign assessments, did Piya Jordan have any adverse reactions to the blood transfusions? Explain.

3. Of the manifestations listed below and on the next page, which are among those associated with a hemolytic transfusion reaction? Select all that apply.

_____ Hypothermia

_____ Chills

_____ Apprehension

_____ Headache

_____ Nausea

_____ Low back pain

_____ Chest pain

_____ Bradycardia

_____ Tachypnea

_____ Hypotension

_____ Hypertension

4. What manifestations are consistent with an allergic transfusion reaction? What type of patient is most likely to experience an allergic transfusion reaction.

5. How can you determine that Piya Jordan did not have a febrile reaction if she was febrile at the beginning of the transfusion?

6. What signs and/or symptoms would you expect to see if Piya Jordan had circulatory overload?

- Click on **Return to Nurses' Station**.
- Click on **Chart** and then on **403** to access Piya Jordan's chart.
- Click on **Expired MARs**.

7. What other blood product has she received since admission? (*Hint:* Look at Tuesday's MAR.)

8. How does this product differ from red blood cells (RBCs), and why was it given to Piya Jordan? (*Hint:* Look at the History and Physical to determine the reason for giving it.)

9. How does administration of this product differ from the administration of RBCs?

Lumbosacral Back Pain

Reading Assignment: Overview of Professional Nursing Concepts for Medical-Surgical Nursing (Chapter 1)
Care of Patients with Problems of the Central Nervous System:
The Spinal Cord (Chapter 43)

Patient: Jacquline Catanazaro, Room 402

Goal: To utilize the nursing process to competently care for a patient with an intervertebral disk problem.

Objectives:

1. Describe the pathophysiology of low back pain.
2. Identify clinical manifestations related to low back pain and/or a herniated intervertebral disk.
3. Plan appropriate interventions to treat low back pain.
4. Evaluate a patient's potential to comply with a health care management plan.
5. Develop an individualized teaching plan for a patient with low back pain.

In this lesson you will learn the essentials of caring for a patient experiencing chronic low back pain. You will explore the patient's history, evaluate presenting symptoms and treatment, plan appropriate nursing interventions to treat the patient's symptoms, and develop an individualized discharge teaching plan. Jacquline Catanazaro is a 45-year-old female admitted with an acute exacerbation of asthma.

Exercise 1

Writing Activity

10 minutes

1. Describe the underlying pathophysiology of low back pain.

2. What differentiates acute low back pain from subacute back pain and chronic low back pain?

3. Match each of the procedures with its correct description.

Procedure	Description
_____ Diskectomy	a. Chips of bones grafted between the vertebrae for support and to strengthen the back; performed after repeated laminectomies or when the spine is unstable; provides stabilization of affected area
_____ Laminectomy	
_____ Spinal fusion (arthrodesis)	
	b. Removal of herniated disk
_____ Percutaneous endoscopic discectomy (PED)	c. Involves microscopic surgery through 1-inch incisions; allows easier identification of anatomic structures, improved precision in removing small fragments, and decreased tissue trauma and pain
_____ Microdiskectomy	
_____ Laser-assisted laparoscopic lumbar diskectomy	d. Removal of part of the laminae and facet joints to obtain access to the disk space
_____ Laser thermodiskectomy	e. Done in combination with percutaneous lumbar diskectomy to shrink the herniated disk; outpatient procedure
	f. Use of special cutting tool threaded through an endoscope for removal or destruction of disk pieces that are compressing the nerve root
	g. Combines a laser with modified standard disk instruments inserted through the laparoscope using an umbilical incision; may be used to treat herniated disks that are bulging but do not involve the vertebral canal

Exercise 2

Virtual Hospital Activity

45 minutes

- Sign in to work at Pacific View Regional Hospital for Period of Care 3. (*Note:* If you are already in the virtual hospital from a previous exercise, click on **Leave the Floor** and then on **Restart the Program** to get to the sign-in window.)
- From the Patient List, select Jacquline Catanazaro (Room 402).
- Click on **Go to Nurses' Station**.
- Click on **Chart** and then on **402**.
- Click on **History and Physical**.

1. According to the History of Present Illness section, what are the patient's complaints in regard to her back? What factors might be contributing to her pain?

2. How does the physician describe this problem under Past Medical History? How was this diagnosed?

3. What is the most common location for a herniated disk? (*Hint:* See Chapter 43 in your textbook.)
   a. L1-2
   b. L2-3
   c. L3-4
   d. L4-5

4. What treatments have been used to manage Jacquline Catanazaro's back pain?

5. Explain the mechanism of action and/or rationale for the treatments Jacquline Catanazaro received 12 months ago.

- Click on **Nursing Admission**.

6. What risk factors does Jacquline Catanazaro have for low back pain and/or herniated disk disease?

7. What assessments should be completed on this patient related to her back pain?

- Click on **Nurse's Notes**.

8. How have the nurses addressed Jacquline Catanazaro's complaint of low back pain?

9. What interventions could you suggest that would be appropriate for this patient's situation?

- Click on **History and Physical**.

10. What is the physician's plan regarding this patient's back pain? What type of interventions might be offered by this consult?

11. If Jacquline Catanazaro's pain is not relieved by nonsurgical management, which of the procedures defined in your clinical preparation would you expect to be used for her? Why?

- Click on **Patient Education**.

12. What goals related to Jacquline Catanazaro's back pain would you add?

13. Develop a discharge teaching plan for her to help relieve and prevent further back pain.

- Click on **History and Physical**.

14. What may interfere with Jacquline Catanazaro's compliance to health care instructions?

- Click on **Return to Nurses' Station**.
- Click on **402** at the bottom of the screen.
- Click on **Patient Care** and then on **Nurse-Client Interactions**.
- Select and view the video titled **1540: Discharge Planning**. (*Note:* Check the virtual clock to see whether enough time has elapsed. You can use the fast-forward feature to advance the time by 2-minute intervals if the video is not yet available. Then click again on **Patient Care** and on **Nurse-Client Interactions** to refresh the screen.)

15. What is your obligation as a health care professional regarding Jacquline Catanazaro's inability to safely manage her care? (*Hint:* See Chapter 1 in your textbook.)

Glaucoma

Reading Assignment: Assessment of the Eye and Vision (Chapter 46)
Care of Patients with Eye and Vision Problems (Chapter 47)

Patient: Clarence Hughes, Room 404

Goal: To utilize the nursing process to competently care for patients with glaucoma.

Objectives:

1. Describe the pathophysiology of glaucoma.
2. Identify clinical manifestations related to glaucoma.
3. Describe appropriate pharmacologic treatment of glaucoma.
4. Administer eye drops safely and accurately.
5. Evaluate a patient's ability to correctly administer prescribed ophthalmic medication.

In this lesson you will learn the essentials of caring for a patient diagnosed with glaucoma. You will explore the patient's history, evaluate presenting symptoms and treatment, administer prescribed medications, and develop an individualized discharge teaching plan. Clarence Hughes is a 73-year-old male admitted for an elective left knee arthroplasty.

Exercise 1

Writing Activity

15 minutes

1. Describe the pathophysiology of glaucoma.

2. Match each description with the type of glaucoma.

Description		Type of Glaucoma
_____	Also known as *acute glaucoma*	a. Primary open-angle glaucoma
_____	Clinical signs include seeing halos around lights and loss of peripheral vision	b. Primary angle-closure glaucoma
_____	Most common form of glaucoma	
_____	Caused by forward displacement of the iris	
_____	Sudden onset of symptoms	

3. Match each diagnostic assessment with its correct description. (*Hint:* Refer to Chapter 46 in your textbook.)

Diagnostic Assessment

_____ Tonometry

_____ Perimetry

_____ Gonioscopy

_____ Ultrasonic imaging of the retina and optic nerve

Description

a. Determines whether POAG or PACG is present. Uses a special lens that eliminates the corneal curve. Is painless and allows visualization of the angle where the iris meets the cornea.

b. Measures the intraocular pressure (IOP). Normal IOP is 10 to 21 mm Hg. A reading of 22 to 32 mm Hg occurs in POAG. PACG can cause IOP readings to exceed 30 mm Hg.

c. Used for patients with ocular hypertension or who are at risk for glaucoma from other problems. Uses computerized programs to assess the thickness and contours of the optic nerve for changes that indicate damage as a result of high IOP.

d. Used to screen visual fields. During this computerized test, the patient is asked to look straight ahead and then indicate, by pressing a control button, when a moving light enters the peripheral vision.

Exercise 2

Virtual Hospital Activity

45 minutes

- Sign in to work at Pacific View Regional Hospital for Period of Care 3. (*Note:* If you are already in the virtual hospital from a previous exercise, click on **Leave the Floor** and then on **Restart the Program** to get to the sign-in window.)
- From the Patient List, select Clarence Hughes (Room 404).
- Click on **Go to Nurses' Station**.
- Click on **Chart** and then on **404**.
- Click on **History and Physical**.

1. What problem of the eye does Clarence Hughes have?

2. How would this problem be diagnosed?

3. What signs and symptoms do you think Clarence Hughes had before being diagnosed?

4. What clinical manifestation should you now assess for related to this diagnosis?

5. The History and Physical does not identify the type of glaucoma Clarence Hughes has. Based on his history and the information in your textbook, which type do you think he mostly likely has? Explain why you came to this conclusion.

- Click on **Return to Nurses' Station**.
- Click on **MAR** and then on **404** to access the correct record.

6. Clarence Hughes has been prescribed two medications to treat his glaucoma. Identify the drug category

   for each medication: Timolol maleate is a _____-_____ _____.

   Pilocarpine is a _____ _____. (*Hint:* See Chart 47-5 in textbook.)

7. Before administering the timolol maleate ophthalmic drops, the nurse should ask Clarence Hughes about any history of comorbidities that may be affected by the medication. Identify what conditions he should be asked about and the rationale for asking.

8. What range of IOP would Clarence Hughes have had before beginning treatment for glaucoma? What would you expect his reading to be during treatment?

- Click on **Return to Nurses' Station**.
- Click on **Chart** and then on **404** for Clarence Hughes' chart.
- Click on **Patient Education**.

9. What educational goals would you add for Clarence Hughes related to his glaucoma?

10. What teaching would you provide to this patient regarding his glaucoma?

11. What would you teach Clarence Hughes regarding his administration of eye drops.

12. What teaching methods would you use to teach medication administration to this patient?

13. How would you evaluate Clarence Hughes' understanding of correct application?

14. If his ophthalmic medications would fail to maintain IOP within normal limits, what other therapy might Clarence Hughes expect to undergo?

LESSON 18

Osteoporosis

Reading Assignment: Care of Patients with Musculoskeletal Problems (Chapter 50)

Patient: Patricia Newman, Room 406

Goal: To utilize the nursing process to competently care for patients with osteoporosis.

Objectives:

1. Describe the pathophysiology of osteoporosis.
2. Assess the patient for clinical manifestations of osteoporosis.
3. Describe appropriate pharmacologic therapy for prevention and/or treatment of osteoporosis.
4. Administer medications safely and accurately.
5. Plan appropriate interventions to promote health and prevent further bone loss in a patient with osteoporosis.
6. Develop an individualized teaching plan for an assigned patient with osteoporosis.

In this lesson you will learn the essentials of caring for a patient diagnosed with osteoporosis. You will explore the patient's history, evaluate presenting symptoms and treatment, and develop an individualized discharge teaching plan. Patricia Newman is a 61-year-old female admitted with pneumonia and a history of emphysema.

Exercise 1

Writing Activity

15 minutes

1. Match each term below with its corresponding definition.

Term	Definition
_____ Bone mineral density (BMD)	a. Bone-building activity
	b. Bone-resorption activity
_____ Osteoblastic	
	c. Low bone mass; T-score is at –1 and above –2.5
_____ Osteoclastic	
	d. The number of standard deviations above or below the average BMD for young, healthy adult
_____ T-score	
_____ Osteopenia	e. Determines the bone strength and peaks between 25 and 30 years of age

2. Describe the pathophysiology of osteoporosis.

3. Describe the different classifications of osteoporosis, including generalized (primary and secondary) and regional.

4. Which medication(s) is (are) associated with the development of osteoporosis? Select all that apply.

_____ Corticosteroids

_____ Antiepileptic drugs

_____ Antihypertensive medications

_____ Thyroid hormone

_____ Cytotoxic agents

_____ Thiazide diuretics

5. What are the most common sites for osteoporosis?

6. At what age should assessments of calcium and vitamin D levels begin?
    a. 35 years
    b. 40 years
    c. 45 years
    d. 50 years

Exercise 2

Virtual Hospital Activity

35 minutes

- Sign in to work at Pacific View Regional Hospital for Period of Care 2. (*Note:* If you are already in the virtual hospital from a previous exercise, click on **Leave the Floor** and then on **Restart the Program** to get to the sign-in window.)
- From the Patient List, select Patricia Newman (Room 406).
- Click on **Go to Nurses' Station**.
- Click on **Chart** and then on **406**.
- Click on **History and Physical**.

1. How long has Patricia Newman been diagnosed with osteoporosis?

2. What risk factors does Patricia Newman have for osteoporosis? Are any of these risks modifiable? If so, which ones?

3. What diagnostic test would have most likely been ordered to diagnose Patricia Newman's osteoporosis? Describe the test and the result that would indicate osteoporosis.

- Click on **Laboratory Reports**.

4. Are any of Patricia Newman's laboratory test results consistent with a diagnosis of osteoporosis?

5. What other laboratory tests might be useful to evaluate Patricia Newman's osteoporosis? Explain the relationship between these tests and bone mineral density.

• Click on **Nursing Admission**.

6. Are there any other risk factors found here? If so, what?

7. What clinical manifestation of osteoporosis is documented on this form?

8. For what other clinical manifestations would you assess Patricia Newman in relation to osteoporosis?

- Click on **Return to Nurses' Station**.
- Click on **MAR** and then on **406** for the correct records.

9. Identify the medications ordered to treat or prevent the worsening of Patricia Newman's osteoporosis. List each medication, along with its order, drug classification, mechanism of action, and frequent side effects. (*Hint:* Consult the Drug Guide if needed.)

10. If you were to administer the prescribed estradiol medication to Patricia Newman, how and where would you apply it? Are there any precautions you should take while applying this?

Exercise 3

Virtual Hospital Activity

35 minutes

- Sign in to work at Pacific View Regional Hospital for Period of Care 3. (*Note:* If you are already in the virtual hospital from a previous exercise, click on **Leave the Floor** and then on **Restart the Program** to get to the sign-in window.)
- From the Patient List, select Patricia Newman (Room 406).
- Click on **Go to Nurses' Station**.
- Click on **Chart** and then on **406**.
- Click on **Patient Education**.

1. What educational goals already identified could be applied to this patient's osteoporosis?

2. What teaching would you provide Patricia Newman regarding exercise to prevent further bone loss? What other exercises might benefit her?

3. What dietary needs does Patricia Newman have related to osteoporosis? What foods would you teach her to include in her diet?

4. Document the teaching points you would review with Patricia Newman regarding the medications prescribed to treat her osteoporosis. (*Hint:* Consult the Drug Guide.)

5. Consider this scenario: Patricia Newman asks you what further treatment would be available if her bone loss continued despite her present regimen. How would you answer her? (*Hint:* Identify five other drug classifications that might be useful to this patient and describe their mechanisms of action.)

6. What is Patricia Newman most at risk for related to her osteoporosis?

7. What can you teach her that would help prevent this from occurring at home?

- Click on **Return to Nurses' Station**.
- Click on **406** to enter Patricia Newman's room.
- Click on **Patient Care** and then on **Nurse-Client Interactions**.
- Select and view the video titled **1500: Discharge Planning**. (*Note:* Check the virtual clock to see whether enough time has elapsed. You can use the fast-forward feature to advance the time by 2-minute intervals if the video is not yet available. Then click again on **Patient Care** and on **Nurse-Client Interactions** to refresh the screen.)

8. Although this discussion was related to Patricia Newman's pulmonary disease, how would smoking cessation benefit her musculoskeletal problem?

9. What other health care disciplines might be useful to help Patricia Newman with her discharge needs related to osteoporosis?

10. What psychosocial nursing diagnosis might be a potential problem for Patricia Newman related to her slightly stooped posture and going home on oxygen? What nursing interventions would be appropriate to help the patient with this difficulty?

Osteomyelitis

_____

Reading Assignment: Care of Patients with Musculoskeletal Problems (Chapter 50)

Patient: Harry George, Room 401

Goal: To utilize the nursing process to competently care for patients with osteomyelitis.

Objectives:

1. Describe the pathophysiology of osteomyelitis.
2. Assess an assigned patient for clinical manifestations of osteomyelitis.
3. Describe the causative agent and category of osteomyelitis in an assigned patient.
4. Safely administer IV antibiotic therapy as prescribed for osteomyelitis.
5. Evaluate diagnostic tests related to osteomyelitis.
6. Develop an individualized discharge plan of care of a patient with osteomyelitis complicated by other disease processes and homelessness.

In this lesson you will learn the essentials of caring for a patient diagnosed with osteomyelitis. You will explore the patient's history, evaluate presenting symptoms and treatment, administer prescribed medications, and develop an individualized discharge teaching plan. Harry George is a 54-year-old male admitted with infection and swelling of his left foot, as well as a history of type 2 diabetes, alcohol abuse, and nicotine addiction.

Exercise 1

Writing Activity

10 minutes

1. Describe the pathophysiology of osteomyelitis.

2. Match each category of osteomyelitis with its correct etiologic description.

Category of Osteomyelitis	Etiologic Description
_____ Chronic	a. Caused by infectious organisms carried by the bloodstream from other areas of infection in the body
_____ Contiguous	
_____ Endogenous/hematogenous	b. Caused by misdiagnosed or inadequately treated infection
_____ Exogenous	c. Caused by infectious organisms entering from outside the body, such as through an open fracture
	d. Caused by skin infection of adjacent tissues

3. What is the most common causative agent of osteomyelitis?
   a. Group A streptococcus
   b. Group B streptococcus
   c. *Staphylococcus aureus*
   d. *E. coli*

4. _____ Older adults with osteomyelitis will often manifest with higher temperatures than other populations with the infection. (True or False)

Exercise 2

Virtual Hospital Activity

45 minutes

- Sign in to work at Pacific View Regional Hospital for Period of Care 1. (*Note:* If you are already in the virtual hospital from a previous exercise, click on **Leave the Floor** and then on **Restart the Program** to get to the sign-in window.)
- From the Patient List, select Harry George (Room 401).
- Click on **Go to Nurses' Station**.
- Click on **Chart** and then on **401**.
- Click on **History and Physical**.

1. Identify the clinical manifestations of local and systemic osteomyelitis below. Using the History and Physical, place an asterisk by any symptoms manifested in Harry George.

   Local

   Systemic

2. Based on what you have read, identify the source of Harry George's osteomyelitis and the type (category) of invasion responsible for it. Explain the rationale for your conclusion.

3. What factors in Harry George's history may have contributed to the development of osteomyelitis? (*Hint:* See Chapter 50 in your textbook.)

- Click on **Physician's Orders**.

4. The following diagnostic tests are useful in the diagnosis and evaluation of osteomyelitis. Match each test with its corresponding description.

Diagnostic Test	**Description**
_____ Magnetic resonance imaging (MRI)	a. Used to determine causative organism
_____ Blood culture	b. Identifies most cases of osteomyelitis
_____ White blood cell count (WBC)	c. Elevated results of this test indicate infection
_____ X-ray of affected extremity	d. Radiologic test that is more sensitive than traditional bone scanning in the diagnosis of osteomyelitis
_____ Radionuclide bone scan	e. Changes with this test do not appear early in the course of the disease
_____ Erythrocyte sedimentation rate (ESR)	f. May be normal early in disease course but rises and remains elevated for up to 3 months after drug therapy is discontinued

5. The most common tool used to assess bone mineral density (BMD) is

_____.

6. Which of the tests listed in the previous question were ordered for Harry George? Which tests were not ordered?

Tests ordered

Tests not ordered

• Click on **Diagnostic Reports**.

7. Identify the results of the tests listed below and compare the results with the pathophysiology of osteomyelitis as described in your textbook. List any documented findings consistent with osteomyelitis and explain what they mean.

Findings documented on the x-ray report

Findings documented on the bone scan

Meaning of both

- Click on **Return to Nurses' Station**.
- Click on **MAR** and select tab **401** for Harry George's records.

8. Determine what routine medications (excluding the continuous IV and insulin coverage) you will be giving to Harry George during the day shift (0700-1500). Below, list the medications you need to give, the drug classification, the reason why each drug is given, and the time each is due. (*Hint:* You may refer to the Drug Guide by returning to the Nurses' Station and then clicking on the **Drug** icon in the lower left corner of the screen. Also see Chapter 50 in your textbook.)

9. Which medication was Harry George receiving that was discontinued on Tuesday? Include dose, route, and frequency.

- Click on **Return to Nurses' Station**.
- Click on **Chart** and then on **401**.
- Click on **Physician's Orders**.

10. What replaced the medication you identified in the previous question? Include dose, route, and frequency.

- Click on **Physician's Notes**.

11. Why was this change ordered?

- Click on **Return to Nurses' Station**.
- Click on **Medication Room**.
- Click on **IV Storage**.
- Click on the **Small Volume** bin and select the medication that you identified in question 9.

12. Review the label for the selected medication. What dilution of this IV antibiotic is available for you to administer?

13. Over what amount of time should you infuse the IV antibiotic? (*Hint:* You may refer to the Drug Guide for this information.)

- Click on **Close Bin** and then on **View Medication Room**.
- Click on **Nurses' Station**.
- Click on **Chart**; then click on **401**.
- Click on **Laboratory Reports**.

14. You are aware that antibiotics have been ordered for Harry George because of his leg infection. You decide to check the WBC results. Document the WBC results for Monday at 1500 and Tuesday at 1100. Compare the results against normal values and indicate whether Harry George's values are normal, elevated, or decreased. Finally, explain the meaning of these results. (*Hint:* Refer to your laboratory reference.)

Total WBC

Neutrophil segs

Neutrophil bands

Lymphocytes

Monocytes

Eosinophils

Basophils

Meaning of the results

- Click on **Return to Nurses' Station**.
- Click on **Patient List**.
- Click on **Get Report**.

15. Read the report. Is there anything else you wish the nurse would have included in the report regarding osteomyelitis? If so, what?

Exercise 3

Virtual Hospital Activity

40 minutes

- Sign in to work at Pacific View Regional Hospital for Period of Care 2. (*Note:* If you are already in the virtual hospital from a previous exercise, click on **Leave the Floor** and then on **Restart the Program** to get to the sign-in window.)
- From the Patient List, select Harry George (Room 401).
- Click on **Go to Nurses' Station**.
- Click on **401** at the bottom of your screen.
- Click on **Take Vital Signs**.

1. Below, record the vital sign findings you obtained.

   BP

   SpO$_2$

   Temp

   HR

   RR

   Pain

- Click on **Patient Care** and then on **Physical Assessment**.
- Click on **Lower Extremities**.

2. Complete a focused neurovascular assessment related to osteomyelitis and document your findings below.

- Click on **Patient Care** and then on **Nurse-Client Interactions**.
- Select and view the video titled **1120: Wound Management**. (*Note:* Check the virtual clock to see whether enough time has elapsed. You can use the fast-forward feature to advance the time by 2-minute intervals if the video is not yet available. Then click again on **Patient Care** and on **Nurse-Client Interactions** to refresh the screen.)

3. How does the nurse describe the progress of Harry George's wound condition? How does the patient respond?

4. Based on your findings from questions 1 through 3, identify three priority nursing diagnoses for Harry George.

- Click on **Medication Room**.
- Click on **MAR** to determine what medications you need to administer to Harry George during this time period (1115-1200).
- Click on **Return to Medication Room**.
- Click on **IV Storage**.
- Click on **Small Volume** and choose the IV antibiotic that is due to be given at 1200.
- Click on **Put Medication on Tray** and then on **Close Bin**.
- Click on **View Medication Room**.
- Click on the **Drug** icon in the lower left corner of the screen.

5. Which IV antibiotic is due to be administered?

6. What is Harry George's dosage for the medication identified in the previous question?

7. What is the recommended dosage for this medication? (*Hint:* See Drug Guide.)

8. Harry George's admission weight was 66 kg. Is his prescribed dosage within the recommended range for dosing?

9. Harry George's physician has ordered peak and trough levels. What is their purpose?

- Click on **Return to Medication Room**.
- Click on **Nurses' Station**.
- Click on **Chart** and then on **401**.
- Click on **Laboratory Reports**.

10. What are Harry George's most recent peak and trough levels?

11. Based on these results, what should your nursing actions be?

12. For what toxic side effects related to nephrotoxicity, neurotoxicity, and ototoxicity must you monitor? (*Hint:* Consult the Drug Guide.)

13. What types of follow-up diagnostic tests should be anticipated for Harry George to determine how well the osteomyelitis is responding to therapy? What changes will occur in these diagnostic test results if therapy is effective?

14. If Harry George's infection does not respond to the antibiotic therapy, what other interventions would most likely be planned? Explain how these would benefit him.

15. Based on what you know and have read, what do you expect will be included in Harry George's discharge instructions and follow-up care to manage his osteomyelitis?

16. Based on Harry George's current living conditions, how do you think his care might best be managed?

Intestinal Obstruction/ Colorectal Cancer

Reading Assignment: Care of Patients with Noninflammatory Intestinal Disorders
(Chapter 56)

Patient: Piya Jordan, Room 403

Goal: To utilize the nursing process to competently care for patients with noninflammatory intestinal disorders.

Objectives:

1. Correlate a patient's history and clinical manifestations with a diagnosis of intestinal obstruction.
2. Evaluate laboratory and diagnostic test results of a patient admitted with a noninflammatory intestinal disorder.
3. Plan appropriate nursing interventions for a patient with a nasogastric (NG) tube.
4. Prioritize nursing care for a patient with an intestinal obstruction.
5. Provide appropriate psychosocial interventions for a patient and family diagnosed with colon cancer.
6. Formulate an appropriate patient education plan for a postoperative patient with colorectal cancer (CRC).

In this lesson you will learn the essentials of caring for a patient admitted with an intestinal obstruction and diagnosed with colorectal cancer. You will explore the patient's history, evaluate presenting symptoms and treatment, plan appropriate nursing interventions, and develop an individualized teaching plan. Piya Jordan is a 68-year-old female admitted with nausea and vomiting for several days following weeks of poor appetite and increasing weakness.

Exercise 1

Writing Activity

20 minutes

1. Describe the pathophysiology of an intestinal obstruction as well as the associated fluid and electrolyte imbalances.

2. Compare and contrast a mechanical and nonmechanical intestinal obstruction.

   a. Mechanical obstruction

   b. Nonmechanical obstruction

3. How does the removal of polyps help to prevent colorectal cancer? (*Hint:* Describe the relationship between polyps and cancer development.)

4. From the list below, select the five most likely sites of metastasis for colorectal cancer. (*Hint:* See Chapter 56 in your textbook.)

_____ Kidney

_____ Brain

_____ Liver

_____ Lungs

_____ Stomach

_____ Adrenal glands

_____ Bone

_____ Thyroid

Exercise 2

Virtual Hospital Activity

40 minutes

- Sign in to work at Pacific View Regional Hospital for Period of Care 1. (*Note:* If you are already in the virtual hospital from a previous exercise, click on **Leave the Floor** and then on **Restart the Program** to get to the sign-in window.)
- From the Patient List, select Piya Jordan (Room 403).
- Click on **Go to Nurses' Station**.
- Click on **Chart** and then on **403**.
- Click on **Emergency Department**.

1. What was Piya Jordan's primary diagnosis according to the Emergency Department record?

- Click on **History and Physical**.

2. What history of symptoms is recorded?

- Click on **Laboratory Reports**.

3. Document Piya Jordan's admission (Monday 2200) results below. Evaluate whether each of the results is normal, decreased, or increased. Provide your rationale for any abnormalities. (*Hint:* Consult your lab manual.)

   Sodium

   Potassium

   Creatinine

   BUN

   Amylase

- Click on **Diagnostic Reports**.

4. What was the result of Piya Jordan's kidney-ureter-bladder (KUB) scan?

5. Why was a computed tomography (CT) scan of the abdomen ordered? What was the result?

6. What part of the bowel is the terminal ileum?

7. Was Piya Jordan's obstruction mechanical or nonmechanical? Explain.

8. If Piya Jordan had sought medical attention before the obstruction worsened, what other diagnostic testing might she have undergone? Explain what that test would show.

- Click on **History and Physical**.
- Click on **Nursing Admission**.

9. Now that you know Piya Jordan has a colonic mass, let's look at her presenting symptoms again. Common clinical manifestations of colorectal cancer are listed below. Which of these signs and symptoms are consistent with Piya Jordan's history and/or physical examination findings on admission? Select all that apply.

_____ Incomplete evacuation

_____ Blood in stool

_____ Narrowing of stools

_____ Change in stool

_____ Straining to pass stools

_____ Anemia

_____ Fatigue

_____ Palpable mass

_____ Pain

_____ Abdominal distention

• Click on **Physician's Orders**.

10. What IV fluid did the Emergency Department physician initially order on Monday at 2115? Why? (*Hint:* Review Piya Jordan's vital signs in the Emergency Department documentation and relate these to fluid/electrolyte changes noted with intestinal obstruction.)

11. What else did the Emergency Department physician order on Tuesday at 0015 to treat the intestinal obstruction? Explain the purpose of this intervention.

• Click on **Return to Nurses' Station**.
• Click on **403** at the bottom of your screen.
• Click on **Patient Care** and then on **Physical Assessment**.

12. Perform a focused abdominal assessment. Document your findings below.

13. Describe any additional assessments and/or interventions that you might do for Piya Jordan related to the intervention identified in question 11.

Exercise 3

Virtual Hospital Activity

45 minutes

- Sign in to work at Pacific View Regional Hospital for Period of Care 3. (*Note:* If you are already in the virtual hospital from a previous exercise, click on **Leave the Floor** and then on **Restart the Program** to get to the sign-in window.)
- From the Patient List, select Piya Jordan (Room 403).
- Click on **Go to Nurses' Station**.
- Click on **Chart** and then on **403**.
- Click on **History and Physical**.

1. Below is a list of risk factors for CRC. Which are documented in Piya Jordan's record? Select all that apply.

   _____ History of polyps

   _____ High-fat, low-fiber diet

   _____ Inflammatory bowel disease

   _____ Age (over 50 years)

   _____ Family history

- Click on **Laboratory Reports**.

2. Below, record Piya Jordan's admission hemoglobin (Hgb) and hematocrit (Hct) from Monday at 2200 and interpret the results. Provide a rationale for any abnormality. (*Hint:* Consult your lab manual.)

   Hgb

   Hct

- Click on **Expired MARs**.

3. What was administered preoperatively to clean out Piya Jordan's bowel?

4. If Piya Jordan's surgery had not been an emergency, describe the type of bowel prep you might have expected to administer. Why is this done?

- Click on **Surgical Reports**.

5. Look at the operative report. Name and describe the surgical procedure.

6. If the tumor had been larger, what further surgery might Piya Jordan have needed? (*Hint:* See Table 56-1 in your textbook.)

7. What is the most likely cell type for Piya Jordan's cancer?

8. How will the physician know what kind of cancer the tumor is?

9. What is the most common type of staging used in colorectal cancer?

10. The treatment of Piya Jordan's cancer will be based on the _____ staging of the disease.

• Click on **Laboratory Results**.

11. Why did the physician order amylase, lipase, and liver function tests? What do the results demonstrate?

• Click on **Return to Nurses' Station**.
• Click on **403** at the bottom of the screen.
• Click on **Patient Care** and then on **Nurse-Client Interactions**.
• Select and view the video titled **1500: Preventing Complications**. (*Note:* Check the virtual clock to see whether enough time has elapsed. You can use the fast-forward feature to advance the time by 2-minute intervals if the video is not yet available. Then click again on **Patient Care** and on **Nurse-Client Interactions** to refresh the screen.)

12. What nursing interventions are discussed during this brief video? Why are they appropriate for Piya Jordan?

- Select and view the video titled **1540: Discharge Planning**. (*Note:* Check the virtual clock to see whether enough time has elapsed. You can use the fast-forward feature to advance the time by 2-minute intervals if the video is not yet available. Then click again on **Patient Care** and on **Nurse-Client Interactions** to refresh the screen.)

13. Piya Jordan's daughter seems to be overwhelmed by her mother's illness and needs. What psychosocial interventions could the nurse plan to help the patient and her daughter? (*Hint:* See Chapter 56 in your textbook.)

14. What would you teach the daughter regarding health promotion and preventing colon cancer in herself?

15. Describe an appropriate teaching plan for Piya Jordan before her discharge.

Malnutrition/Obesity

Reading Assignment: Care of Patients with Malnutrition: Undernutrition and Obesity
(Chapter 60)

Patients: Harry George, Room 401
Jacquline Catanazaro, Room 402
Piya Jordan, Room 403

Goal: To utilize the nursing process to competently care for patients with nutritional disorders.

Objectives:

1. Identify patients at risk for malnutrition.
2. Perform a nutritional screening assessment on assigned patients.
3. Evaluate laboratory findings in relation to a patient's nutritional status.
4. Plan appropriate dietary interventions for a patient with malnutrition.
5. Identify a patient's risk factors related to obesity.
6. Formulate an appropriate patient education plan for an overweight patient.

In this lesson you will learn the essentials of caring for patients with nutritional disorders. You will explore the patient's history, perform a nutritional screening assessment, evaluate findings, and plan appropriate nursing interventions, including each patient's educational needs. Harry George is a 54-year-old male with a 4-year history of type 2 diabetes admitted with infection and swelling of his left foot. Piya Jordan is a 68-year-old female admitted with nausea and vomiting for several days following weeks of poor appetite and increasing weakness. Jacquline Catanazaro is a 45-year-old female admitted with an acute exacerbation of asthma.

Exercise 1

Writing Activity

5 minutes

1. The 2015-2020 Dietary Guidelines for Americans emphasizes the need to focus on what?
   a. Variety, nutrient density, and amount
   b. Adding calories from saturated fat
   c. Increasing non-weight-bearing exercise
   d. Eating a vegetarian diet

2. The USDA's MyPlate recommends that half of each meal should consist of _____

   and _____.

3. When providing education to a vegan, a nurse must remember that this group is at an increased risk for a deficiency of which vitamin?
   a. Vitamin B_1
   b. Vitamin B_2
   c. Vitamin B_6
   d. Vitamin B_{12}

Exercise 2

Virtual Hospital Activity

40 minutes

- Sign in to work at Pacific View Regional Hospital for Period of Care 1. (*Note:* If you are already in the virtual hospital from a previous exercise, click on **Leave the Floor** and then on **Restart the Program** to get to the sign-in window.)
- From the Patient List, select Harry George (Room 401) and Piya Jordan (Room 403).
- Click on **Go to Nurses' Station**.
- Click on **Chart** and then on **401** for Harry George's record.
- Click on **History and Physical**.

1. What risk factors for malnutrition are noted in Harry George's History and Physical?

- Click on **Return to Nurses' Station**.
- Click on **Chart** and then on **403** for Piya Jordan's record.
- Click on **History and Physical**.

2. What risk factors for malnutrition are noted in Piya Jordan's History and Physical?

3. According to your textbook, an evaluation of a patient's nutritional status should include what seven areas?

- Click on **Return to Nurses' Station**.
- Click on **401** to enter Harry George's room.
- Click on **Patient Care** and then on **Physical Assessment**.

4. Using Harry George's documented height and weight on admission, calculate his body mass index (BMI).

- Click on **Laboratory Reports**.

5. Harry George's albumin level is _____ g/dL.

6. Based on your findings, is Harry George malnourished or at risk for malnutrition? Explain how you came to your conclusion.

Exercise 3

Virtual Hospital Activity

40 minutes

- Sign in to work at Pacific View Regional Hospital for Period of Care 1. (*Note:* If you are already in the virtual hospital from a previous exercise, click on **Leave the Floor** and then on **Restart the Program** to get to the sign-in window.)
- From the Patient List, select Harry George (Room 401) and Piya Jordan (Room 403).
- Click on **Go to Nurses' Station**.
- Click on **403** to enter Piya Jordan's room.
- Click on **Patient Care** and then on **Physical Assessment**.

1. Calculate Piya Jordan's BMI based on her current height and weight.

2. Piya Jordan's albumin level is _____ g/dL.

3. Evaluate the results of your findings. Is Piya Jordan malnourished or at risk for malnutrition? Explain how you came to your conclusion.

4. Compare and contrast your findings for Harry George and Piya Jordan. What are the similarities? What are the differences?

5. Is the serum albumin level the best indicator of a patient's nutritional status? What other laboratory tests would give you more information on Piya Jordan's and Harry George's nutritional status?

6. Identify two nursing diagnoses related to the malnourished status of these two patients.

7. What type of diet or dietary supplements would you recommend for these two patients?

Exercise 4

Virtual Hospital Activity

30 minutes

- Sign in to work at Pacific View Regional Hospital for Period of Care 2. (*Note:* If you are already in the virtual hospital from a previous exercise, click on **Leave the Floor** and then on **Restart the Program** to get to the sign-in window.)
- From the Patient List, select Jacquline Catanazaro (Room 402).
- Click on **Go to Nurses' Station**.
- Click on **Chart** and then on **402**.
- Click on **Nursing Admission**.

1. Record Jacquline Catanazaro's current height and weight below.

2. Calculate her BMI.

3. Based on her BMI, is Jacquline Catanazaro's nutritional status normal, overweight, obese, or morbidly obese?

- Click on **History and Physical**.

4. What complication of obesity does Jacquline Catanazaro suffer from?

5. What other complications is she at risk for?

6. What are the contributing factors for her increased weight?

- Click on **Return to Nurses' Station**.
- Click on **MAR** and then on **402**.

7. Do any of the medications ordered for Jacquline Catanazaro cause weight gain? If so, explain below. (*Hint:* Return to the Nurses' Station and consult the Drug Guide.)

- Click on **Return to Nurses' Station** and then on **402** to enter Jacquline Catanazaro's room.
- Click on **Patient Care** and then on **Nurse-Client Interactions**.
- Select and view the video titled **1140: Compliance—Medications**. (*Note:* Check the virtual clock to see whether enough time has elapsed. You can use the fast-forward feature to advance the time by 2-minute intervals if the video is not yet available. Then click again on **Patient Care** and on **Nurse-Client Interactions** to refresh the screen.)

8. What concern does the patient voice regarding her medications?

9. Evaluate the nurse's response. Was it appropriate? Was it accurate? Explain.

10. What else could the nurse have suggested to help this patient lose weight?

11. If diet and exercise alone do not work for Jacquline Catanazaro, what other treatment options might she have?

Diabetes Mellitus, Part 1

Reading Assignment: Care of Patients with Diabetes Mellitus (Chapter 64)

Patient: Harry George, Room 401

Goal: To utilize the nursing process to competently care for patients with diabetes mellitus.

Objectives:

1. Describe the pathophysiology of diabetes mellitus.
2. Compare and contrast the characteristics of type 1 and type 2 diabetes.
3. Identify the relationship between diabetes and other disease processes.
4. Evaluate a patient's risk factors for diabetes.
5. Assess a patient for short- and long-term complications of diabetes.
6. Develop an appropriate plan of care for a patient with type 2 diabetes.

In this lesson you will learn the essentials of caring for a patient admitted with complications related to diabetes mellitus. You will explore the patient's history, evaluate presenting symptoms and treatment, plan appropriate nursing interventions, and develop an individualized teaching plan. Harry George is a 54-year-old male with a 4-year history of type 2 diabetes admitted with infection and swelling of his left foot.

Exercise 1

Writing Activity

20 minutes

1. Describe the pathophysiology of diabetes mellitus and the basis for the resulting abnormalities in carbohydrate, protein, and fat metabolism.

2. Briefly define and summarize the etiologic differences between type 1 and type 2 diabetes mellitus.

3. Provide the distinguishing features of type 1 diabetes mellitus (DM) for each of the features below.

Former names

Age at onset

Symptoms

Antigen patterns

Antibodies

Endogenous insulin
and C-peptides

Nutritional status

Inheritance

Insulin

Medical nutrition therapy

4. Provide the distinguishing features of type 2 DM for each of the features below.

Former names

Age at onset

Symptoms

Antigen patterns

Antibodies

Endogenous insulin
and C-peptides

Nutritional status

Inheritance

Insulin

Medical nutrition therapy

Exercise 2

Virtual Hospital Activity

45 minutes

- Sign in to work at Pacific View Regional Hospital for Period of Care 1. (*Note:* If you are already in the virtual hospital from a previous exercise, click on **Leave the Floor** and then on **Restart the Program** to get to the sign-in window.)
- From the Patient List, select Harry George (Room 401).
- Click on **Go to Nurses' Station**.
- Click on **Chart** and then on **401**.
- Click on **History and Physical**.

1. What risk factors for diabetes are noted in Harry George's history?

2. Describe the history of his present illness.

3. What is the relationship between the infection in Harry George's foot and his diabetes mellitus?

- Click on **Laboratory Reports**.

4. Harry George's blood glucose level on admission was _____ mg/dL.

5. What abnormalities in his urinalysis results can be attributed to diabetes? Explain the relationship.

- Click on **Emergency Department**.

6. What factor in Harry George's recent history most likely contributed to his hyperglycemia? (*Hint:* Read the Emergency Department physician's notes for 1345.)

- Click on **Nursing Admission**.

7. Listed below are clinical manifestations of diabetes mellitus identified in the textbook. For each manifestation, indicate (with Yes or No) whether it is usually present in type 2 diabetes.

   Polyuria

   Polydipsia

   Polyphagia

   Visual blurring

   Fatigue

   Weight loss

   Chronic complications

8. To what extent does Harry George fit the typical picture of a patient with type 2 diabetes mellitus?

- Click on **Return to Nurses' Station**.
- Click on **401** to enter Harry George's room.
- Click on **Patient Care** and then on **Nurse-Client Interactions**.
- Select and view the video titled **0735: Symptom Management**. (*Note:* Check the virtual clock to see whether enough time has elapsed. You can use the fast-forward feature to advance the time by 2-minute intervals if the video is not yet available. Then click again on **Patient Care** and on **Nurse-Client Interactions** to refresh the screen.)

9. What does Harry George tell the nurse about his appetite?

10. What diet has been ordered for this patient? (*Hint:* Review his chart.)

11. Describe the principles of this diet.

12. How might the patient's alcohol intake affect his blood glucose levels?

Exercise 3

Virtual Hospital Activity

40 minutes

- Sign in to work at Pacific View Regional Hospital for Period of Care 2. (*Note:* If you are already in the virtual hospital from a previous exercise, click on **Leave the Floor** and then on **Restart the Program** to get to the sign-in window.)
- From the Patient List, select Harry George (Room 401).
- Click on **Go to Nurses' Station**.
- Click on **Chart** and then on **401**.
- Click on **Physician's Orders**.

1. What test is ordered that can be used to determine Harry George's control of diabetes mellitus? Describe the purpose of this test. How often should it be done?

- Click on **Laboratory Reports**.

2. What were the results of this test for Harry George? Based on these results, evaluate and explain how well his diabetes is controlled.

3. What implication does Harry George's level of glycemic control have for his future?

- Click on **Return to Nurses' Station**.
- Click on **401** at the bottom of the screen.
- Click on **Patient Care** and then on **Physical Assessment**.

4. Perform a head-to-toe assessment on Harry George. Document any abnormal results below.

Head & Neck

Chest

Back & Spine

Upper Extremities

Abdomen

Pelvic

Lower Extremities

- Click on **EPR** and **Login**.
- Choose **401** from the Patient drop-down menu and **Neurologic** from the Category drop-down menu.

5. Below, document any abnormal information obtained from the neurologic assessment completed on Monday at 1835.

- Select **Cardiovascular** from the Category drop-down menu.

6. Below, document any abnormal information obtained from the cardiovascular assessment completed on Monday at 1835.

7. Describe the following potential long-term complications for diabetes mellitus.

Cardiovascular disease

Cerebrovascular disease

Retinopathy (nonproliferative and proliferative)

Peripheral vascular disease

Neuropathy

Nephropathy

Erectile dysfunction

8. Does Harry George exhibit signs or symptoms that would alert you to the possibility of any of the long-term complications noted in question 7? If so, explain.

9. What interventions, including patient teaching, would you plan to offer Harry George for prevention of injury secondary to reduced sensation in his left foot? (*Hint:* See Chart 64-6 in your textbook.)

LESSON 23

Diabetes Mellitus, Part 2

Reading Assignment: Care of Patients with Diabetes Mellitus (Chapter 64)

Patient: Harry George, Room 401

Goal: To utilize the nursing process to competently administer medications prescribed to treat patients with diabetes mellitus.

Objectives:

1. Describe the pharmacologic therapy used for a patient with diabetes.
2. Evaluate a patient's response to insulin therapy.
3. Assess a patient for side effects of insulin therapy.
4. Describe the clinical manifestations of hypoglycemia as a side effect of insulin therapy.
5. Develop an individualized teaching plan for a patient with type 2 diabetes.

In this lesson you will learn the essentials regarding pharmacologic therapy for a patient admitted with complications related to diabetes mellitus. You will identify, describe, administer and evaluate effects of prescribed antidiabetic medications. Harry George is a 54-year-old male with a 4-year history of type 2 diabetes. He was admitted with infection and swelling of his left foot.

Exercise 1

Writing Activity

30 minutes

1. Match each insulin to its appropriate classification. (*Note:* Classifications may be used more than once.)

Insulin	**Classification**
_____ Isophane insulin NPH injection (Humulin N, Novolin N)	a. Rapid-acting
_____ Human lispro injection (Humalog)	b. Short-acting
_____ Insulin glargine injection (Lantus)	c. Intermediate-acting
_____ Regular human insulin injection (Humulin R, Novolin R)	d. Long-acting
_____ Insulin aspart (Novolog)	

2. Which insulin has the quickest onset of action?
   a. Humulin N
   b. Humulin R
   c. Levimir
   d. Novolog

3. Which insulin has no identifiable peak effect?
   a. Humalog
   b. Lantus
   c. Novolin N
   d. Toujeo

4. Which insulin has the longest duration of action?
   a. Humulin 70/30
   b. Relion N
   c. Tresiba U-100
   d. Humulin R U-500

5. Match each classification of oral hypoglycemic agents to its appropriate mechanism of action.

Classification

_____ Alpha glucosidase inhibitors

_____ Amylin analogs

_____ Biguanides

_____ DPP-4 inhibitors

_____ Incretin mimetics (GLP-1 agonists)

_____ Insulin sensitizers

_____ Insulin stimulators (secretagogues)

_____ Sodium glucose transport inhibitors

Mechanism of Action

a. Trigger release of insulin from the beta cells

b. Act like natural gut hormones to decrease glucagon and glucose secretion and delay gastric emptying

c. Delay digestion of starches and the absorption of glucose from the small intestine

d. Decrease liver glucose production and improve sensitivity of insulin receptors

e. Prevent an enzyme from breaking down natural gut hormones, allowing for decreased glucagon secretion and glucose production

f. Inhibit glucose production by the liver, inhibit intestinal absorption of glucose, and increase insulin sensitivity

g. Decrease endogenous glucagon, delay gastric emptying, and trigger satiety

h. Prevent kidney reabsorption of glucose and sodium

6. Match each medication with its appropriate classification. (*Note:* Classifications may be used more than once.)

Medication

_____ Arcabose

_____ Canagliflozin

_____ Glipizide

_____ Glimeperide

_____ Liraglutide

_____ Metformin

_____ Pioglitazone

_____ Pramlintide

_____ Repaglinide

_____ Sitagliptin

Classification

a. Alpha glucosidase inhibitor

b. Amylin analog

c. Biguanide

d. DPP-4 inhibitor

e. Incretin mimetic

f. Insulin sensitizer

g. Insulin stimulator

h. Sodium glucose transport inhibitor

Exercise 2

Virtual Hospital Activity

40 minutes

- Sign in to work at Pacific View Regional Hospital for Period of Care 1. (*Note:* If you are already in the virtual hospital from a previous exercise, click on **Leave the Floor** and then on **Restart the Program** to get to the sign-in window.)
- From the Patient List, select Harry George (Room 401).
- Click on **Go to Nurses' Station**.
- Click on **Chart** and then on **401**.
- Click on **Emergency Department**.

  1. What two medications were ordered to control Harry George's diabetes? Include the dose and route for each.

  2. How would you give the IV insulin? (*Hint:* You can access the Drug Guide by clicking on the **Drug** icon in the lower left corner of the screen in the Nurses' Station.)

  3. Find the Emergency Department physician's progress notes for Monday at 1345. What does the physician plan to order for the sliding scale insulin coverage?

- Click on **Physician's Orders**.

  4. Look at the orders for Monday at 1345. What was the actual sliding scale insulin order?

- Click on **Return to Nurses' Station**.
- Click on **Kardex** and then on **401** to access the correct record.

5. According to the Kardex, how often should the capillary blood glucose be tested?

- Click on **Return to Nurses' Station**.
- Click on **MAR** and then on **401** for Harry George's records.

6. According to the MAR, when should the insulin sliding scale be administered? What was the time of this order?

7. What would you do regarding the inconsistencies identified above?

8. What problems might occur if Harry George does not receive insulin at bedtime?

- Click on **Return to Nurses' Station**.
- Click on **401** at the bottom of the screen.
- Click on **Clinical Alerts**.

9. What is the clinical alert for 0730?

Prepare and administer the sliding scale insulin for this glucose level by following these steps:

- Click on **Medication Room** on the bottom of the screen.
- Click on **MAR** or on **Review MAR** at any time to verify how much insulin to administer based on sliding scale. (*Hint:* You may click on **Review MAR** at any time to verify correct medication order. You must click on the correct room number within the MAR. Remember to look at the patient name on the MAR to make sure you have the correct patient's records. Click on **Return to Medication Room** after reviewing the correct MAR.)
- Click on **Unit Dosage** and then on drawer **401** for Harry George's medications.
- Select **Insulin Regular**, put medication on tray, and then close the drawer.
- Click on **View Medication Room**.
- Click on **Preparation** and choose the correct medication to administer. Click on **Prepare**.
- Click on **Next**, choose the correct patient to administer this medication to, and click on **Finish**.
- You can click on **Review Your Medications** and then on **Return to Medication Room** when ready. Once you are back in the Medication Room, you may go directly to Harry George's room by clicking on **401** at the bottom of the screen.
- Click on **Patient Care**.
- Click on **Medication Administration** and follow the steps in the Administration Wizard to complete the insulin administration.

10. How much insulin should be administered?

11. What is the preferred site of administration for fastest absorption?

12. List the expected onset, peak, and duration for the insulin you just administered. What actual times would you expect the onset, peak, and duration for Harry George, based on giving the insulin at 0730?

    Onset

    Peak

    Duration

13. At what time would Harry George be at most risk for hypoglycemia? Describe the signs and symptoms that would indicate this acute complication.

14. While you are preparing to administer Harry George's insulin, he asks you why he is taking this because he did not use insulin at home. How would you answer this?

15. For what side effects should you monitor Harry George related to his insulin regimen?

Exercise 3

Virtual Hospital Activity

35 minutes

- Sign in to work at Pacific View Regional Hospital for Period of Care 4. (*Note:* If you are already in the virtual hospital from a previous exercise, click on **Leave the Floor** and then on **Restart the Program** to get to the sign-in window.)
- Click on **Chart** and then on **401** for Harry George's chart. (*Remember:* You are not able to visit patients or administer medications during Period of Care 4. You are able to review patient records only.)
- Click on **Nurse's Notes**.

1. Read the notes for Wednesday at 1730. What does the patient say regarding glyburide?

2. How would you respond to the patient's demands?

3. How often did Harry George take the glyburide at home?

4. Why do you think the oral regimen was increased in the hospital? What concerns might you have regarding this increase? (*Hint:* This patient is also receiving insulin.)

5. What classification of oral hypoglycemic does glyburide belong to? (*Hint:* For help, click on the **Drug Guide** located on the counter in the Nurses' Station.)

6. For what side effects of glyburide should you assess Harry George?

7. What specific patient teaching points should you give this patient regarding glyburide?

- Click on **EPR**.
- Select **401** from the Patient drop-down menu and **Vital Signs** from the Category drop-down menu.
- Click on **Exit EPR**.
- Click on **Chart** and then on **401**.

8. List the date and time, blood glucose levels, and insulin doses received since Harry George's admission. (*Hint:* There are eight. You will need to access the chart and review the expired MARs to obtain the sliding scale doses.)

9. Based on Harry George's pattern of blood glucose levels, would you evaluate his current therapy as effective? If not, how might the physician further treat his diabetes?

10. If you were reviewing the chart orders and the EPR on Wednesday evening and found the information recorded in the table in question 8, what would you be ethically and legally bound to report?